LIVING WITH M.E.

LIVING WITH M.E.

Dr. Charles Shepherd

CEDAR

An imprint of William Heinemann Limited

Published by Cedar
an imprint of William Heinemann Limited
Michelin House, 81 Fulham Road, London SW3 6RB

LONDON MELBOURNE AUCKLAND

Copyright © 1989 Charles Shepherd
First published in Great Britain 1989
Reprinted 1989 (twice)

0 434 11165 2

Photoset by Rowland Phototypesetting Limited
Bury St Edmunds, Suffolk
Printed and bound in Great Britain by
Cox & Wyman Ltd, Reading, Berks.

To my wife, Pam, who has stuck by me through all the difficult times.

Contents

Acknowledgement

I should like to acknowledge the help of Dr Melvin Ramsay, who diagnosed my own illness back in 1982.

Dr Ramsay was the consultant physician in infectious diseases at the Royal Free Hospital, London, at the time of the outbreak of M.E. there in 1955. He has done more than anyone else to keep interest in M.E. to the fore. Without his dogged determination to establish proper recognition and diagnostic criteria for M.E., the scientific evidence to support his theories might never have come to light, and the entire medical profession would still regard the illness as being 'just in the mind'.

Foreword

There is still a great deal of confusion in the mind of the medical profession regarding the precise clinical identity of myalgic encephalomyelitis and this can, in great measure, be attributed to the current belief that M.E. and the many post-viral fatigue states are synonymous. Far from being synonymous they are distinguishable, in the first place, by the long delay in the restoration of muscle power after even a minor degree of physical effort; secondly, by the extraordinary variability of symptoms even in the course of one day; and finally, by the alarming tendency of the disease to become chronic. On the other hand, the fatigue factor in the post-viral states is merely part of a general fatigue, shows no daily variability and the condition is unlikely to last longer than two years.

The incidence of M.E. among doctors is out of all proportion to their numbers in the general population. Dr Charles Shepherd has now had the disease for close on ten years. His experience of the vagaries of the disease – alternating periods of remission and relapse since the diagnosis was confirmed in 1982 – puts him in an ideal position to help other victims of this distressing complaint.

The chronic M.E. sufferer faces a condition of constant muscle fatigue, often severe muscle pain and discomfort as a result of spasm and twitchings. This is accompanied by cerebral dysfunction in the form of impairment of memory and powers of concentration, emotional lability, disturbed sleep rhythm, vivid dreams, and lack of muscle co-ordination that renders the patient incapable of carrying out simple manoeuvres. This is all too often accompanied by a sense of rejection by friends and relatives as a hopeless neurotic. Dr Shepherd can give these pitiful victims of a disease that is still imperfectly understood, invaluable assistance in the planning of their lives, on a basis that can afford them a sense of purpose in combating what would otherwise be a drab and pointless existence. I thoroughly commend his excellent treatise.

Dr A. Melvin Ramsay
President of the Myalgic Encephalomyelitis Association

Introduction

It is often said that doctors have no real understanding of a disease unless they contract it themselves. I have been suffering from M.E. for the past ten years and so have first-hand experience of its debilitating symptoms and of the havoc it can wreak on both career and family life. All thoughts of running my own general practice in the country have had to be abandoned; my wife has become chief breadwinner in addition to shouldering most of the responsibility for running our home and bringing up two young children; M.E. has imposed severe limitations on our lives. Incapacitating though it is, M.E. is only now coming to be recognised by the medical profession as a genuine disease. So, what is it like to have M.E.?

Imagine waking up every single morning for months, even years, with the certain knowledge that for the rest of the day you will be wandering around feeling as though you have flu; that your brain will soon become fogged and completely unable to function correctly, and that after even a short walk to the shops you may be forced to lie down feeling exhausted. Not a very pleasant thought, but that's what it's like having M.E. M.E. not only reduces your day to a few useful hours in which you may be able to function with some degree of normality, it can actually take years out of a whole lifetime.

M.E. is short for myalgic encephalomyelitis, which simply means an illness affecting the muscles (myalgia = muscle pain), the brain (encephalo) and the nervous tissue (myelitis). The cardinal features of the disease are muscle fatigue induced by exercise and brain malfunction, which follow on in the aftermath of an acute flu-like viral infection, often in a previously fit young adult. These muscle and brain symptoms, although chronic and sometimes lasting for months and even years, will vary in their severity throughout the day, and from day to day – something not seen in any other illness where fatigue is a major feature.

Despite these highly characteristic features, many M.E. patients still visit doctors who don't recognise the disease and who regard their symptoms with great scepticism. Patients who complain of being 'tired all the time' (known as 'TATT' in medical shorthand), along with a seemingly endless list of other unrelated symptoms constitute a considerable diagnostic problem. So, unless fully aware of the symptoms of M.E., a doctor may not make the right diagnosis, which means that patients are offered inappropriate advice.

Despite all the recent publicity, M.E. is not a 'new disease'. Outbreaks of the illness have been reported in Europe, America, Australia and New Zealand on a regular basis for the past fifty years, and it is now estimated that there are 100,000 sufferers in the U.K. alone. In the early days research into M.E. was hampered by the lack of facilities available for identifying 'culprit' viruses; today it is believed that the group of viruses to which polio belongs (the enteroviruses) is likely to be the major cause of the disease. Following the initial infection – which may take the form of flu or gastric enteritis – it seems that a susceptible individual is unable to kill off the virus, which persists in the bowel, then multiplies and passes via the bloodstream to invade the nerve and muscle cells. Why this should be so remains a mystery, but factors such as physical and mental stress during the acute illness are probably quite important.

In addition, the persisting virus could be stimulating excessive production of substances like interferon and interleukin, the body's natural immunising chemicals, which are normally released only in the acute stage of a viral illness. So it could be that both the persisting virus and the immune chemicals are affecting the way muscles, brain and nerves are able to carry out their normal functions.

As yet, there is no drug that will 'cure' M.E., or significantly alter the natural course of the disease. The recent research findings, and the tremendous interest being shown by scientists in other persisting infections (e.g. AIDS) may well open up the way to specific forms of therapy in the near future.

Rest, both physical and mental, is at present the key aspect to recovery from M.E., and this will involve sufferers and their families in having to make some very significant changes in lifestyle. Patients have to learn to 'listen to their bodies' and to live within their limitations – not very easy advice to take, particularly for previously fit and active young adults.

M.E. patients can and do make a significant – or full – recovery, even after long periods of time, so never give up hope. The aim of my book is to give sufferers and those caring for them all the information about the disease currently available. Armed with this information I hope you will be better equipped to make the right choices in how to manage your individual case of M.E., and to give your body the optimum conditions for a slow but progressive recovery.

Charles Shepherd

PART 1:
WHAT IS M.E.?

1. First Appearances

THE ROYAL FREE DISEASE

In the late spring of 1955 the infectious diseases unit at the Royal Free Hospital in London began admitting patients from all over north London with an infection that had doctors baffled.

Initially the illness was unremarkable, with respiratory symptoms, sore throat, enlarged lymph glands and a slight fever. Some patients also had a gastric upset and a few had marked dizziness (vertigo). Then, instead of getting progressively better, new symptoms started to appear – headaches, blurred or even double vision (diplopia) and abnormal sensations in the skin (paraesthesiae). All the patients had difficulties with brain functioning, particularly with short-term memory and concentration, but the most striking feature of the disease was the severity of muscle fatigue caused by even the most limited exercise. The patients also had cold hands and feet, were troubled by bladder disturbances and were extremely sensitive to any change in external temperatures.

The doctors at the Royal Free were in no doubt: these patients had an infection that the body's front line of defence – the lymphatic glands – seemed unable to filter out, and it was spreading to the nerves and muscles. However, no such illness had been clearly defined in the textbooks.

The degree of muscle weakness the patients complained of initially suggested polio – still a possibility in those days – but there was no muscle wasting taking place, which is one of polio's most characteristic features. Other investigations failed to confirm the presence of polio, so the doctors were left with an infection looking for a cause.

Some patients were given an EEG (electroencephalogram) to measure their brain activity. A few did show abnormalities, and an assumption was made that they were experiencing some form of brain inflammation (encephalitis) and that the cause was a virus, but not the polio virus.

Then the most dramatic events of that year occurred, involving the Royal Free's own medical and nursing staff. The virus broke out at the hospital on 13 July, and over the following twelve days seventy doctors and nurses were taken ill. So many staff became involved that the hospital was forced to close, and it remained closed until 5 October. In all there were 292 cases, but very significantly only twelve of the hospital's patients – who were resting in their beds – fell victim to the disease.

Just like the cases admitted earlier, the hospital staff's illness followed the characteristic pattern of symptoms we now associate with M.E. First came the non-specific flu-like illness with the sort of symptoms that can occur in any viral infection. Following this acute onset some of the staff – now patients themselves – had a short period of remission in which they began to get a little better. Then it became obvious that their defence mechanisms had not limited the spread of the virus after all, and that it had passed through this 'safety net' to reach brain, nerves and muscles. The patients started to feel ill again with the characteristic features of brain malfunction, nervous disturbances and overwhelming muscular fatigue.

Unlike most of the patients we see with M.E. today, many of those involved at the Royal Free had definite abnormalities in their nerves, which could be demonstrated on clinical examination. At the Royal Free nearly 20 per cent of the patients had a paralysis of the facial nerve – the one which controls our facial expressions – and eleven had paralysis of swallowing, and even had to be tube-fed. Clinical examination showed that the nervous system had been affected by the disease in 74 per cent of patients.

Two other important features of the disease that emerged from this outbreak were the pain and sensory changes experienced by some of the sufferers. Doctors found that the slightest movement of one of the weakened limbs could result in severe pain, and there was often pain too below the ribs which coincided with extreme tenderness in the corresponding muscles. Other patients had significant areas where the skin sensation was lost (hypoaesthesiae); in some cases this involved half the body. Twenty-eight of these cases were investigated with electromyograms (EMG), which show how messages are transmitted from the brain via the nerves to the muscles. The results suggested that there were definite abnormalities in the way these messages were being carried.

The dramatic way in which this mystery disease paralysed a whole hospital made it headline news, and the papers called it 'the Royal Free disease'. But the inconclusive nature of the tests, which failed to isolate the cause of the epidemic, left many members of the medical profession sceptical, and they lost interest in further research. Some of the patients quickly got better, but others have remained permanently disabled. One person who did not forget their plight was Dr Melvin Ramsay, consultant physician in the infectious diseases unit. He published a report in *The Lancet* on some of the cases at the Royal Free the year after the outbreak, in which a leading article described the disease as 'A New Clinical Entity?', and suggested it be named 'benign myalgic encephalomyelitis'. The term 'benign', implying that M.E. is not a serious or fatal condition, has with hindsight been dropped, but myalgic encephalomyelitis remains the most common name for the disease.

What happened at the Royal Free made the disease briefly famous, but there have been other less spectacular outbreaks – over seventy in fact – reported worldwide, particularly in affluent countries with temperate climates. Outbreaks seem to occur more frequently in closed communities such as schools, hospitals and barracks, where an infectious disease can spread quickly; however, it must be emphasised that though a viral infection can be caught from another person, susceptibility to that infection persisting and turning into M.E. is not something that can be passed on. It should also be noted that M.E. is an endemic disease, meaning that there are individual cases occurring all the time, as well as periodic small outbreaks that present in specific geographic localities.

OTHER OUTBREAKS OF M.E. IN BRITAIN

In 1952 an infectious disease, never identified, but which sounds remarkably like M.E., broke out at the Middlesex Hospital in London. In 1955, just before the Royal Free outbreak, there was a cluster of cases with classic M.E. symptoms at a primary school in Cumbria in the north of England. A small outbreak in a teacher training college in Newcastle-upon-Tyne occurred in 1959. The cases here supported the theory that – as with polio – physical stress during the acute infection was an important co-factor in the development of M.E. The student teachers shared their accommodation with a group of nuns; the students developed M.E., but the nuns, who were naturally leading a very quiet life, did not.

During 1964–6 a large number of cases was reported from the north London practice of Dr Betty Scott, who made the interesting observation that many of her patients had low blood sugars (hypoglycaemia), which may turn out to be important in view of the disordered energy metabolism now being demonstrated in some patients' muscles.

One further outbreak of interest in Britain occurred during 1970–1 at London's Great Ormond Street Children's Hospital. Once again those affected were mainly the nursing staff, and none of the children who were patients on the wards at the time succumbed. There were nearly 150 cases in all. The Great Ormond Street nurses had a list of almost identical symptoms to those experienced at the Royal Free, and again went on to follow the by now familiar pattern of remission followed by relapse or continuing disability.

More recently, during the early 1980s, outbreaks along with sporadic cases have been reported in the medical journals from several parts of Scotland. Here, virologists have at last been able to link M.E. with one specific sub-group of enteroviruses – Coxsackie B – which means that one of the most important parts of the M.E. jigsaw has started to fit into place.

M.E. IN THE U.S.A.

In America the condition is variously referred to as epidemic neuromyasthenia, chronic mono, chronic Epstein-Barr virus disease, the chronic fatigue syndrome or 'Yuppie Flu'.

The first ever recorded outbreak of M.E. in the United States involved doctors and nurses at the Los Angeles County General Hospital in 1934. At first the disease was thought to be polio, but although the patients' muscles remained weak they did not become wasted, so this explanation had to be ruled out. Altogether nearly 200 members of staff were affected, and when they were thoroughly reviewed six months later half were still unwell. Further small outbreaks continued to be reported from various parts of the U.S., but the American public did not really become aware of the condition until 1985, when following an outbreak at Lake Tahoe, Nevada, media attention became overwhelming. There was a general demand that action should be taken, and a proper research programme be initiated.

The shores of Lake Tahoe are a retreat for successful, active, professional 'high achievers' – the last type of person to stay away from work without good reason. Late in 1984 strange things started happening in the area – previously fit adults in their thirties and forties started falling ill with a mysterious flu-like illness which was then followed by the classic muscular fatigue and intellectual malfunction associated with M.E. So many people were involved that the press got interested and one magazine labelled the area 'Raggedy Ann Town', as the sufferers said they felt like Raggedy Ann dolls. The local doctors were initially quite baffled by the illness. All the tests were coming back normal, and they began to have doubts as to whether the patients had a physical illness at all. Perhaps, against all the odds, the sufferers were just work-shy.

Fortunately, two doctors, Dan Peterson and Paul Cheney, did not share these doubts; they became increasingly convinced that the steady stream of patients arriving at their consulting rooms were genuinely ill. They decided it was time to get to the bottom of the mystery. Their patients had sore throats, glandular swellings and headaches, and they wondered if this might be glandular fever (called in America infectious mononucleosis). The problem was that glandular fever is a teenage disease: patients in the age group affected should have developed antibodies and be immune to the virus by now. Nevertheless, the similarity with glandular fever led Peterson and Cheney to research into the Epstein–Barr virus (EBV), which causes it.

The Epstein–Barr virus belongs to the herpes group of viruses, which cause cold sores, genital herpes and chickenpox. EBV is passed on from person to person by saliva – hence the term 'kissing disease' for glandular fever. Carriers of the disease can pass it on without developing it themselves. By the age of thirty, nearly 90 per cent of all adults will have developed antibodies to EBV, indicating a full degree of immunity, so after this age an attack of glandular fever becomes very rare.

All the viruses in the herpes group have the capacity to stay on in the body after causing an initial infection, so acting as a reservoir of dormant infection. So once a person has been infected by EBV, the virus does not go away, but remains for life, usually without causing any harm, in the salivary glands and the B cells of the immune system, which are responsible for antibody production. The virus is kept in check by other cells of the immune system known as natural killer cells.

What Doctors Peterson and Cheney began to wonder was whether the Epstein–Barr virus, lying dormant in the B cells, had been reactivated and let loose in the body again to produce the American fatigue syndrome that they were witnessing at Lake Tahoe. In other words was something weakening the body's immune system, which up until now had prevented the dormant virus from becoming active? Was the virus now multiplying, and leaving the B cells to start a further episode of glandular fever, from an original infection which the patients had been harbouring since picking it up as children? After all, other members of the herpes group of viruses can be reactivated from their dormant state, given the right circumstances. Herpes cold sores will reappear at times of stress, during menstruation, in hot sun, or when the patient is feeling run down – exactly the same sort of stimuli now known to cause a relapse or exacerbation of M.E.

Doctors Cheney and Peterson decided to look for evidence of Epstein-Barr virus in the Lake Tahoe patients. They found raised antibodies to EBV in about three-quarters of them, but this still left a quarter with normal levels and a small percentage with no antibodies at all. The hypothesis was further complicated by the fact that EBV antibody tests are difficult to interpret, and that the Lake Tahoe patients produced a fairly similar spread of results that would be expected from a 'normal' group of people of their age. So no conclusions could be drawn to support the EBV theory in Lake Tahoe.

In the meantime the American press and broadcasting media had become extremely interested in the mystery virus, and the outbreak was now receiving extensive publicity throughout the United States. The magazine *Newsweek* referred to it as the 'malaise of the 80s' and other papers used the name 'Yuppie Flu', as so many of the sufferers were fit young professionals. Somewhat prematurely, the name chronic Epstein-Barr disease became the accepted term for the illness, and a national CEBV association was founded in Portland, Oregon. They were soon receiving requests for information from all over the U.S. Numerous individual patients started asking their physicians if CEBV could be the cause for their persisting ill health, and pressure came from Congress for researchers to start finding some answers.

Blood samples were now sent to Dr Robert Gallo, the scientist who had been working on the AIDS virus at the National Cancer Institute and who had recently isolated the first 'new' herpes group virus for twenty years (human herpes virus type 6). The results of his research are awaited with interest, but so far have not turned out to conclusively link one of these herpes viruses.

The Lake Tahoe outbreak eventually subsided, but as in the

outbreaks already described, many of those who were taken ill still have not recovered. About one-third got better, about half followed the familiar pattern of remission and relapse, and the rest remain chronically unwell.

M.E. IN OTHER PARTS OF THE WORLD

Despite increasing recognition of M.E. in Britain and America, doctors in the rest of Europe remain for the most part sceptical that such a disease exists. However, outbreaks have occurred in Switzerland, in 1937 and 1939 at army barracks, and in Iceland in 1948. When the Icelandic patients were re-examined seven years later it was found that of those who had been severely affected only 25 per cent had recovered; of those who had the disease only mildly, still only 44 per cent had got completely better. One interesting fact about this outbreak was that it seemed to have immunised people against polio, because in 1955 an epidemic of polio in Iceland failed to make any impression in the area in which M.E. had taken hold.

In Australia and New Zealand M.E. is taken much more seriously. In Adelaide there was an epidemic of 700 cases of M.E. between 1949 and 1951. New Zealand and New South Wales both saw outbreaks in the early 1980s, and the two countries have their own self-help organisations for sufferers.

In Adelaide there is important research going on into the red blood cells of sufferers. Observed under an extremely high-powered electron microscope these have shown gross abnormalities of shape, no longer resembling the small 'floating doughnuts' that can easily squeeze down minute blood capillaries with their vital supplies of oxygen. Dr Tapen Mukherjee, who made this observation, has noted similar changes in the blood of runners after a marathon – which gives a good idea of the exhaustion many M.E. sufferers feel most of the time.

Most of the important Australian research is being carried out in Sydney at the Prince of Wales–Prince Harry Hospital.

2. What Triggers M.E.?

Following the outbreak of M.E. at the Royal Free Hospital in 1955, Dr Melvin Ramsay was left with many questions to answer. In all the recorded outbreaks the illness seemed to have been triggered by an infection, presumably a virus, which was impervious to attack by the body's immune system. Which virus or viruses were responsible? Did the virus ever go away, even when a patient apparently got better, or did it remain dormant, with the possibility of being reactivated? A lot of research needed to be done into the way the virus affected the patient's brain, nerves and muscles, and hopefully this would produce some answers.

One thing that Dr Ramsay has remained utterly convinced about is that M.E. is a genuine disease, but many of his colleagues continued to be sceptical, so it was not easy persuading specialists in the fields of virology, neurology and immunology to become involved in M.E. research. Fifteen years after the Royal Free outbreak two psychiatrists dealt a severe blow to the credibility of M.E. when they published papers concluding that the disease was purely hysterical in origin. This had a devastating effect on the medical establishment, and M.E. became unfashionable and even unmentionable. Even today, with so much concrete evidence that the disease exists, some doctors persist in accusing M.E. patients of malingering and the controversy still rages.

Nevertheless, the search for a cause of M.E. goes on. No single virus has been identified and U.K. scientists now believe that viruses belonging to the enteroviral group are the prime culprits.

THE ENTEROVIRUSES

Enteroviruses are a group of seventy-two different viruses that can live and multiply in the intestines – hence 'entero'. They often remain there without causing any ill effects, but can occasionally go on to invade other parts of the body, causing a wide range of illnesses that probably include M.E.

Enteroviruses occur all over the world. In tropical countries they are around all through the year; in temperate climates, where M.E. is most prevalent, they flourish mainly during the summer months. Most adults come into contact with at least one, and the result is the sort of symptoms we label as a 'summer cold'. Children in the first few years of life – 'the nappy years' – are much more frequently infected by enteroviruses, and may remain carriers without any ill effects, while being capable of passing the infection on to adults who come in contact with them or their excreta. Most adults will have developed some degree of immunity to enteroviruses, particularly if they have lived in the tropics, where they are often passed on in conditions of overcrowding or poor hygiene.

Enteroviruses can also survive in sewage; so where contaminated waste is disposed of into our seaside estuaries there may be another reservoir of infection for unsuspecting bathers and eaters of seafood. This may be one reason why some people seem to develop M.E. after a seaside holiday, and why pockets of infection are reported from coastal areas where sewage is dumped.

Once inside the body enteroviruses commonly infect the throat, causing tender enlarged glands in the neck. However, there is usually very little in the way of symptoms at all. The fact that the neck glands are swollen means that the virus is being attacked by the body's immune system. The problem occurs if the immune system is not capable of dealing with the virus. Then it can enter the blood and pass to various other tissues where it likes to live. If the virus enters the brain, muscles and nerves, then the patient has M.E.

As time goes by, other parts of the body may become infected, so that the patient develops secondary symptoms that are seemingly unconnected with each other. Such symptoms are

14

often baffling to a doctor who is uninformed about M.E. and may reinforce the view that the patient's illness is 'all in the mind'.

Over the past ten years evidence has slowly accumulated linking M.E. to one particular sub-group of the enteroviruses – the Coxsackie viruses. These Coxsackie viruses (thirty in all) are named after a small town on the Hudson River in New York State, where the virus was originally isolated from an outbreak of polio-like illness. The researchers started off by looking at M.E. patients to see if they had developed any antibodies to Coxsackie viruses in their blood. They looked for two types of specific antibodies. First, an antibody called a neutralising antibody, which tends to persist for a long period of time after the initial infection. Second, for one called IgM antibody, which if present, suggests that the virus is persisting. Although many of the M.E. patients had these two antibodies present, the results are difficult to interpret and cannot be used as a diagnostic test for M.E., as some quite healthy people also carry the same antibodies in their blood.

Professor James Mowbray, at St Mary's Hospital, London, has now developed a more sophisticated blood test (the VP1 test) which can actually identify the presence of any one of the enteroviruses. And for patients in whom the test is negative it is possible that the cause here is the Epstein-Barr virus. He has also developed a method of separating and then culturing (growing) enteroviruses from stool samples, and his initial results show that some M.E. patients definitely have a persisting reservoir of infection present in their intestines.

One more exciting development is the gene probe, a technique devised to test for viral nucleic acid (RNA) in the muscle cells. Dr Len Archard, at Charing Cross Hospital, London, has been looking at muscle biopsies from M.E. patients and testing them with the genetic coding for the specific nucleic acid inside the Coxsackie virus. His results indicate that the virus is present inside about one-quarter of the samples, and some of the others have the Epstein-Barr virus present.

The next question that needs answering is, what is it *doing* in the muscle? It does not seem to be killing the muscle cells or using them as a breeding ground, but it may well be interfering with the genetic apparatus of the muscle cells, somehow 'switching off' their normal function and thus causing a disturbance in energy production.

So now there are several different tests which can help to demonstrate the presence of enterovirus in the body:

- Blood tests for antibodies made against the virus, along with the VP1 test which picks up the actual virus.
- A stool test which can grow the enterovirus.
- Gene probes which can isolate viral genetic material inside cells.

Research into M.E. still has a long way to go, but if the rapid progress of the past few years continues we should soon have some more conclusive answers.

HOW THE BODY'S IMMUNE SYSTEM WORKS

The study of immunology is invaluable to the understanding of M.E. because it seems that the disease may be caused by the continuing failure of the immune system to eradicate the culprit virus.

The body's first line of defence against disease consists of the regional lymph glands, which quickly swell up when an infection occurs within their territory – as they can when you have a sore throat. Antibodies are then produced locally by the lymphatic tissue which pass to the site of infection, such as the lining mucosa of the throat or bowel. Their function is to try to prevent any further spread into the blood stream. Once the virus has produced this localised response a second line of defence is activated and other antibodies are made in the blood. These help to neutralise the virus and stop it spreading to other tissues, such as the muscle and nerves in the case of enteroviruses. These antibodies will also stop any reinfection by remaining active in the blood after the disease has been eradicated.

One further crucial part of the immune system are cells called T lymphocytes, which have important regulatory functions over the immune response. Some of these cells, called T suppressors, can dampen down an immune response. Others, called T helpers, act rather like the conductor of an orchestra and help to co-ordinate all the different specialist cells, as well as stimulating B cells to produce antibodies.

It is these T helper cells which have been shown to be reduced in number in some M.E. patients, and they are also known to be severely affected in illnesses like AIDS where there is a severe deficiency.

Other changes in the immune response, involving excessive production of immune chemicals called lymphokines, are also being observed. In any acute viral infection, the immune system's natural response is to produce these substances, which cause symptoms such as malaise along with general aches and pains. But if the virus then persists, perhaps their production is maintained, and this may be the reason for the continuing 'flu-like feeling of which most M.E. sufferers complain.

Support for this theory comes from work at the Royal Free Hospital, where patients with certain types of liver disease were given interferon as part of their treatment, and then went on to develop some M.E. symptoms as a side effect. *The Lancet* has also reported an outbreak of M.E. amongst children in mid Wales, who were found to be producing excessive interferon.

Dr Peter Behan, in Glasgow, is now looking at raised levels of another immune chemical called interleukin one beta, which is known to have important effects on various tissues and cell functions, but particularly in the hypothalamus, from where many M.E. symptoms may be originating.

THE FIGHT AGAINST VIRUSES

All viruses are made up of two parts. On the outside is a protein-coated capsule, called the capsid, which contains the antigens against which human antibodies are mobilised. Inside there is a core of nucleic acid (the genome) which is the genetic material of the virus. Viruses are classified according to the type of nucleic acid within this core. Some, like the herpes viruses

17

(Epstein–Barr virus, chickenpox) contain DNA (deoxyribonucleic acid). Others, like the enteroviruses contain RNA (ribonucleic acid).

HOW VIRUSES REPLICATE

1 The virus meets the host cell and becomes attached to its outer surface. This is just like a key fitting into a lock, as the virus has to find specific receptors on the surface to fit into. If antiviral antibodies are being made, part of their function is to block these receptor sites (1(b)).

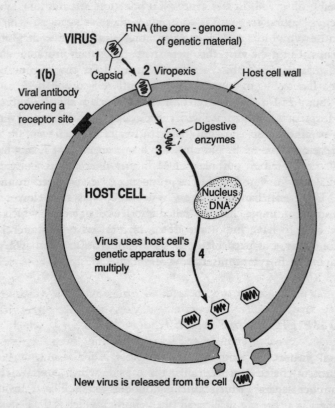

2 The successful virus penetrates the cell wall: this is called viropexis.

3 The capsule or capsid of the virus is stripped off by intra-cellular enzymes, so that its genetic information is freed.

4 The viral nucleic acid (RNA or DNA) then takes over the host cell's own genetic apparatus, using it to manufacture new viral particles. This very complicated process is again controlled by the host cell's own enzymes.

5 The new virus, which has been assembled and recoated by the host cell then passes out through the cell membrane.

During this process the host cell may end up being so damaged that it ceases functioning normally and dies. However, in some cases of persisting infection, where the virus remains dormant (as with Epstein–Barr virus), the cell may not be significantly damaged. Another possibility is that although the virus itself may not be causing any great harm, the patient's immune system may still be reacting against it, and in the process causing cell damage – an autoimmune process. It is this mechanism which has been suggested as a reason for the continual liver damage in someone chronically infected by hepatitis B, and this type of response may just have some relevance in M.E.

Antiviral drugs are not like the broad spectrum antibiotics, which can kill off a whole range of bacterial infections. Because they have to avoid damaging the normal cells invaded by the virus, the aim is to make them act at very specific enzyme-controlled stages, where the virus is using the host cell to replicate itself. The host cell's enzymes behave differently according to whether the invader contains DNA or RNA. Consequently drugs effective against DNA viruses do not work on RNA viruses.

At present there are no antiviral drugs available which are effective against RNA-containing viruses such as the enteroviral group. There is one antiviral drug – Acyclovir – which is effective against some of the DNA-containing herpes viruses, and this drug is proving particularly useful for treating severe cases of chickenpox where there is life-threatening pneumonia or encephalitis, or for shortening the duration of herpetic cold sores.

Acyclovir interferes with the replication of the DNA and has no adverse effect on the host cell. It is only effective in cells containing a herpes virus and once inside acts like a magic bullet in its specificity. The problem is that it only works when the virus is actively multiplying, so although it will help to reduce the severity of an acute attack of cold sores it will not prevent a recurrence once the virus becomes latent within the cell. The possible role of Acyclovir in the management of chronic Epstein-Barr virus infection is still being assessed in America, but there appear to be no clear benefits at present.

Other antiviral drugs directed at other specific viruses are now in the research stage. No doubt in time antiviral drugs for RNA viruses will become available, but their future use in M.E. remains uncertain.

If it is as yet impossible to eradicate culprit enteroviruses, an alternative treatment could be to interfere with the patient's immune response. Immunotherapy, like the development of antiviral drugs, is also, unfortunately for M.E. patients, in its infancy. It used to be very popular to treat the sort of prolonged debility that sometimes followed glandular fever with a short course of high-dose steroids, and some doctors have given these drugs to M.E. sufferers in a desperate attempt to buck them up. As steroids actually dampen down and depress the immune system (they are immunosuppressive), they would now seem to be a very inappropriate choice of drug in M.E.

Other forms of immunotherapy which have recently been tried include the removal of immune complexes (the combined particles of virus and antibody present in the blood) by a process known as plasma exchange, and secondly, the use of a drug called inosine pranobex (Imunovir) which is claimed to stimulate the immune system into producing more T lymphocytes, as well as having some weak antiviral properties. Neither of these two approaches has, as yet, shown any conclusive benefits.

Another form of immunotherapy is the administration of gammaglobulin by injection. This is basically a way of giving M.E. patients a concentrated mixture of natural antibodies. Gammaglobulin is extracted from the plasma of pooled blood that has been donated by thousands of normal healthy people. After having the injections some patients report that they feel much better, although the improvement may last only a short while, so the drug has to be given at regular intervals. Others derive no benefit at all, and a few seem to feel even worse. A properly controlled trial is now under way both in the U.K. and in Australia to assess the value of gammaglobulin injections, and the results should be available shortly.

Future treatment of M.E. using drugs will obviously depend on a greater understanding of the damage being caused in the patient's muscles, nerves and immune system, as well as on the identification of the viruses triggering the illness and the reasons for their persistence. Hopefully one of the large pharmaceutical companies will be prepared to invest time and money on research into more antiviral drugs. It may also be necessary to find a way of limiting the body's production of immune chemicals like interferon and interleukin: at the moment all the effort is going into the production of this type of chemical for therapeutic use.

The advances outlined in this chapter concerning our understanding of M.E. have been very significant. If this progress can now continue over the next few years we could have some specific treatment worth using.

WHO CAN GET M.E.?

M.E. can be contracted by a previously fit man or woman who picks up a common viral infection. When perfectly fit individuals come into contact with a virus, they usually have a short self-limiting illness, with a sore throat and swollen neck glands. They then quickly develop antibodies and produce specific white blood cells that eradicate the virus, and they get better. For reasons not yet fully understood, the immune system in a small minority of individuals fails to kill the virus. It persists, and they go on to develop M.E.

Thus, developing M.E. is not determined solely by picking up a specific virus, but also by the susceptibility of the patient to that virus. Though it is difficult to generalise, a hypothesis is emerging that certain co-factors increase a patient's susceptibility to M.E. Age, sex and the extent of physical and mental stress experienced at the time of catching the infection all seem to play a part in determining whether or not the patient goes on to

M.E.
Possible pathogenesis :

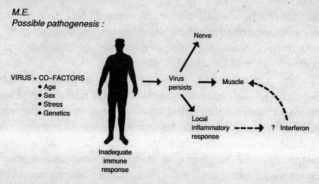

develop M.E. There is a similarity here with polio: patients who exercised while incubating the virus were more likely to suffer a severe attack of the disease.

AGE

Age is an important factor in determining susceptibility to both enteroviruses and the Epstein-Barr virus, so far considered the likely culprits in M.E. Children who come into contact with EBV usually develop no illness at all, just protective antibodies. When infected with enteroviruses, they likewise tend to suffer only minor self-limiting illnesses with no after-effects.

However, the body's immune system reacts in different ways to a variety of infections according to age, and as it matures it does not necessarily increase its protective role. 'Childhood illnesses' like rubella, mumps and measles often affect adults far more severely and for longer than they do the young. Teenagers who have not developed immunity to EBV get glandular fever, which may leave them debilitated for months; it is now suggested that a reactivation of dormant EBV may be responsible for M.E. in some adults. Enteroviral infections can also cause serious diseases in adults, including inflammation of the brain and heart, and may even prove fatal.

The peak age for M.E. seems to be the thirties. It is probably also significant that women of this age are frequently in contact with young children and babies: enteroviruses can be caught from contact with infected faeces. Though about three-quarters of M.E. sufferers first develop their illness at some time between their late teens and early forties, there are also well-documented cases of young children and elderly people being affected.

SEX

There appears to be a strong female bias in M.E. with three or four cases of women getting M.E. to every one male victim. Outbreaks involving female nursing staff have frequently been reported over the years, though in other outbreaks the sex ratio was equal, and there have been a few instances where only men have been affected, for example in the Swiss army barracks. If women *are* predominantly affected, could there be any logical reasons for this?

First, mothers of young children are in constant contact with the very group that acts as a reservoir of enterovirus infection, passing it on in their faeces to susceptible individuals. Teachers and nurses, other groups commonly affected by M.E., are in a similar position.

Second, when women are ill and need to rest, their domestic and family commitments make it very difficult for them to do so. Unless their husbands can take time off work or extra help is drafted in to look after the family, they just cannot rest, no matter how ill they feel.

Third, women are more likely to know about M.E. and so get it diagnosed. Most of the recent publicity for the condition has been in women's magazines. No such information has been specifically aimed at men, so far fewer of them have probably even heard of M.E.

Finally, there is the question of hormones. There is some experimental evidence to support the theory that female hormones can affect the body's immunity, and certainly many women sufferers notice a considerable alleviation of symptoms during pregnancy, when there are very significant shifts in the hormone pattern taking place.

In the laboratory, female mice may die young when introduced to a specific infection, but the males tend to survive. If, however, the sex hormones are removed from the males they will also succumb rapidly, and if the females are given the male sex hormone testosterone their resistance will significantly improve. In scientific experimentation one must be extremely careful about concluding that results from animals will also apply in the same way to human beings. However, these results do give some support to the theory that the sex hormones may be related to the risk of someone acquiring M.E. on meeting the 'right' virus at the right time.

PHYSICAL AND MENTAL STRESS

One of the most significant co-factors in increasing susceptibility to developing M.E. appears to be undue physical or mental stress at the time of the original viral infection. Time and again I hear the same story of conscientious patients who struggle on in some stressful occupation or with family commitments, while feeling absolutely terrible, until they are finally forced to stop through sheer physical and mental exhaustion. Back at the Royal Free outbreak in 1955 it was the doctors and nurses, constantly on their feet, mentally and physically stressed, who were taken ill, while only twelve of the patients who were resting in their beds actually succumbed!

There is also some interesting experimental research to support the theory that exercise can be bad for one's health at the time of an infection. Athletes undergoing strenuous physical training programmes show decreased activity in various aspects of their normal immune response. Compared to a group of similar age, who are not undergoing such vigorous activity, the 'active' group is likely to develop more respiratory infections. There are also disturbing reports, from time to time, of sportsmen actually dying while carrying out vigorous exercise – particularly playing squash – at the time of an acute viral infection. The enterovirus Coxsackie can directly affect the heart muscle at the time of the acute illness, and may be the reason for some of these fatalities. In experiments in the laboratory, if the enterovirus Coxsackie B3 is given to two groups of mice, one exercising and the other living a sedentary existence, the exercising mice are more susceptible to the virus.

There are numerous reports of M.E. patients who, having started to make a degree of recovery, go and participate in some form of vigorous athletic activity. They join in a game of hockey or try a marathon run, only to find that this sudden burst of physical activity has left them completely poleaxed, and now their M.E. has relapsed again after a period of relative remission. This sort of activity is clearly *not* recommended for any M.E. patients – well or unwell – until they have remained in very good health for a considerable period of time, and even then only with great caution.

It is not only physical stress that adversely affects the body's immunity. Mental stress and important 'life events' such as family crises, unemployment, bereavements and serious illness all seem capable of depressing the immune system, not only in the person affected, but also in those who are emotionally close. Any crisis could well help to tip the balance in the way someone copes with a viral infection in the first place, as well as influencing how they cope with the continuing illness.

A WESTERN DISEASE?

It has recently been suggested that in some cases of M.E., especially where there appears to be a gradual onset, the cause may not be a virus at all, but the result of an allergy, or possibly from chemicals and toxins in the environment. This is an attractive theory, but so far there is no real evidence to back it up.

Some scientists are coming round to the idea that environmental pollution, along with the 'Western way of life', with its junk food, additives, cigarettes and excessive alcohol intake, may be steadily weakening the body's immune system over a long period of time. Then, when a particular infection comes along, the immune system has become so overloaded that it can no longer cope, and conditions like M.E. are triggered off.

There is not much evidence for M.E. occurring in non-Westernised societies; maybe it is just not recognised in these parts of the world, but a more likely explanation is the fact that poor public health exposes children to far more enteroviruses, allowing a greater degree of immunity to develop before they reach the 'at-risk' age.

Allergic diseases, particularly hay fever and asthma, appear to increase in incidence when the Western way of life is introduced into primitive communities, so it may be that our environment does play some as yet undefined role in the disease process.

From the information so far gathered, it is still impossible to predict who might develop M.E., and how their particular disease is going to progress. However, the classic 'at risk' patient is female, in her mid-twenties to thirties, and coping with a fair amount of physical and mental stress. The majority of such individuals who contract the 'culprit' virus will *not* develop M.E. All we can say at present is that we have some of the explanations, but we still do not know them all.

WHO CAN RECOVER FROM M.E.?

'Will I ever get better?' is the first question the M.E. patient wants an answer to once the diagnosis has finally been established. Yes, you can recover from M.E.; it may take several years, but it is still possible after even quite long periods of time. Taking strict rest in the very early stages and readjusting lifestyle seem to have the most positive effect on outcome – which is why late diagnosis and inappropriate management can be so harmful. Until all doctors are able to recognise M.E. in its earliest stages, and to offer correct advice, many patients will not be taking the enforced rest they desperately require.

Any patient who makes steady progress during the first year or so of this illness can reasonably expect this to continue into the third and fourth years, although nothing is absolutely certain with M.E. Obviously the longer the condition remains chronic, without any significant progress, the less likely full recovery is.

M.E. is a very individual condition; some of the symptoms will come and go or vary in severity, whereas others will be there for most of the time. Patients will inevitably go through both good and bad periods during the course of this illness, so accurately assessing what will happen in the long term is very difficult.

Some patients want to know if having an acute or gradual onset to their illness affects chances of recovery. At present there are no accurate statistics available, but some doctors feel that those who develop M.E. in a more gradual fashion, with repeated infections producing a slow deterioration in health, may not do quite so well. One doctor researching M.E. wrote recently that most of his patients had improved over a year, and provided they can take adequate rest in the early stages of the disease, this will apply to many sufferers. However, the attitude that the patient should be *better* by the end of a year is mistaken, though unfortunately still quite common among many doctors, who feel that when all you have had is a bit of post-viral debility you really cannot still be ill a whole year later.

The majority of M.E. sufferers tend to fall into three broad groups. Firstly there are the patients who, after months or years, make a full or significant degree of recovery, and so return to their normal pattern of life.

The second group of patients tends to follow a much more erratic course, with periods of remission and relapse. During periods of remission they may return to relative normality, even going back to work and starting to lead a normal social life once again. Then M.E. returns – it may be sudden and precipitated by another infection, or undue stress, or an excessive bout of physical activity. However, a few patients just seem to fall back into ill health for no apparent reason. For some, periods of remission can be shortlived, but I know of other M.E. sufferers who have enjoyed better health for years before succumbing to a relapse. For those whose remissions seem to be getting longer, and their relapses less severe, the eventual outlook is probably quite optimistic.

In the third group are those patients who have chronic unremitting M.E. Dr Melvin Ramsay has described this condition as 'a baffling syndrome with a tragic aftermath'. Follow-up studies of the outbreaks of M.E. described in this book have shown a significant number of patients who remain chronically disabled. Some of the nurses involved in the first recorded outbreak, in Los Angeles in 1934, were thoroughly reviewed nearly fifteen years later and found to be suffering the same muscle fatigue and brain malfunction. They had never managed to return to work. Similarly, over thirty years on from the famous outbreak at the Royal Free Hospital, many of those who were affected remain unwell today.

There is no doubt that some patients with M.E. will have to learn to live with a long-term illness that fluctuates in severity, and to cope with the same difficulties suffered by people with other chronic neurological disorders, like multiple sclerosis. Although some of their symptoms will undoubtedly come and go, and there will be good days to compensate for many of the bad ones, the cardinal features of muscular fatigue and brain malfunction will be present for most of the time. This group of patients will have to accept that life for the foreseeable future is going to be a plateau of ill health interrupted by recurrent exacerbations. The cold months of the year are often a particularly bad time.

Whichever group you seem to fit into, never give up hope. In the meantime accept your limitations, listen to what your body is telling you, and don't try to fight M.E. – it just won't work!

3. M.E. – The Cardinal Symptoms

THE ONSET OF M.E.

For the majority of M.E. patients, the illness tends to follow on in the wake of an acute infection. A previously fit individual contracts a mild and unremarkable flu-like illness – and from that point on the patient never really feels well again. Sometimes the initial illness is specific, as in my own case, where M.E. was triggered by chickenpox, and sometimes it can be traced back to a gastric upset contracted while on holiday, possibly caused by bathing in infected water or eating contaminated seafood. But the initial symptoms of most patients follow a pattern we all recognise from bouts of ordinary flu.

There may be swollen and tender lymph glands in the neck and armpit, along with a slight rise in temperature and some general aches and pains. Some patients complain of an associated gastroenteritis ('gastric flu'), or respiratory symptoms such as a sore throat or cough. Marked dizziness and vomiting are an occasional prominent feature, which may lead the doctor to misdiagnose the illness as labyrinthitis – an infection in the inner ear. Occasionally severe chest pains are reported; patients are sometimes admitted to hospital with a suspected heart attack. The explanation may well be that the enterovirus is affecting either the lining of the heart, causing pericarditis; or the heart muscle itself, causing myocarditis; or that the muscles of the ribcage have become inflamed, which is known as Bornholm's disease. These presentations in M.E. are fairly uncommon but very important, and should not be missed by doctors, as it is now thought that enteroviruses may be one of the commonest causes of infective myocarditis.

As the initial flu-like symptoms start to subside there may be a short period when the patient begins to feel a return to normal. However, most M.E. sufferers continue to feel unwell and tired. As they try to resume a normal life, the cardinal M.E. symptoms of exercise-induced muscular fatigue and brain malfunction become more and more apparent, and any undue stress from an early return to work quickly causes a marked exacerbation.

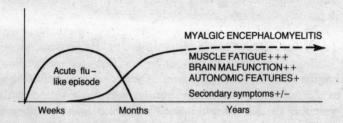

MYALGIC ENCEPHALOMYELITIS
MUSCLE FATIGUE +++
BRAIN MALFUNCTION ++
AUTONOMIC FEATURES +
Secondary symptoms +/−

Acute flu-
like episode

Weeks   Months   Years

Although the majority of patients develop M.E. in this way, a few have an insidious or gradual onset of the disease, where there is no obvious triggering infection. The symptoms seem to develop over a longer period of time with recurrent mild infections, sore throats and swollen glands, resulting in a progressive deterioration in health. It may be that infection with the 'right virus' did initially take place, and that although it caused no obvious bout of illness at the time, it went on to persist in the body, eventually causing the characteristic features of M.E. to appear. These features are muscle fatigue and malfunction of the brain and nerves.

MUSCLE FATIGUE AND PAIN

Exercise-induced muscular fatigue is the cardinal feature of M.E. − if this is not one of your symptoms then the diagnosis is not M.E. Rapid muscular fatigue, particularly in the arms and legs, will follow any physical exertion that the sufferer makes. The load-bearing muscles of the legs are always affected, and many patients notice that the effort of standing still for long periods may be more tiring than going for a walk. If the patient persists in physical activity after fatigue has set in, the result will be weakness and even total exhaustion. The activity involved may be very minimal, such as walking a few hundred yards or doing some light gardening, but for some severely affected M.E. patients even this is too much, and they can find themselves becoming almost housebound.

As M.E. is such an individual illness, different patients have widely varying capabilities as far as their exercise tolerance is concerned, but each sufferer soon learns to recognise his or her limitations and the dangers of exercising beyond such limits. Once the point of fatigue/weakness/exhaustion has been reached the M.E. patient will be forced to stop, rest and recover while energy levels return to normal, just like recharging a battery.

The arm muscles become fatigued and weak after lifting heavy objects or reaching up to put things on to a high shelf. Any repetitive activity using these muscles quickly produces weakness, and even a simple task like washing hair can leave some patients feeling thoroughly exhausted.

The highly characteristic recovery period in M.E., during which the energy starts to return to normal in the muscles, can take minutes, hours, even days – it all depends on the extent to which the sufferer has exceeded his or her capabilities. Exercising to the point of physical exhaustion can result in a very prolonged period of relapse.

Many M.E. patients describe how they have 'tired, aching muscles that wear out easily', and one patient recently described to me how she had spent a considerable part of her life literally crawling around on her hands and knees. A few sufferers notice that their muscle weakness seems to be worse on one side of the body, and this is often the side which they would regard as being their strongest. So, a right-handed person would find that the right side is predominantly affected. In general, though, muscular weakness will occur in any muscle that is being over-used. Even the very small muscles in the eye are affected, so that vision may become blurred after prolonged reading.

M.E. sufferers invariably find it extremely tiring trying to perform physical and mental activities simultaneously. This is partly why teachers, hairdressers and nurses with M.E. can find returning to work so difficult, and why pushing the supermarket trolley round to do the weekly shop can be such a debilitating experience. Equally, any sporting activity that requires concurrent physical and mental activity becomes an impossibility.

Despite enforced inactivity, muscle wasting is unusual in M.E., and it should not occur unless the sufferer has been completely immobile for a considerable period of time.

MUSCULAR PAIN

Muscular pain (myalgia) is a second frequently mentioned muscular symptom of M.E., but not everyone experiences it. Some patients seem to experience a great deal of pain, particularly in tender localised areas such as the neck and back. Others just have general aches or cramps following on after exercise.

Pain in the tendons, which connect the muscles to bones in the joints, may also occur.

The third quite common muscle feature is twitching of the muscles – referred to by doctors as fasciculation. This abnormality can occur in normal people who are run down, but its frequency in M.E. suggests that here it is probably related to the abnormal lack of co-ordination between the nerve messages and the muscle fibres. Fasciculations may just be noticed as ripples under the skin, or they can be quite coarse. They can appear almost anywhere in the body from large muscle groups in the arms and legs to the smaller muscles controlling the eyelids. Involuntary flickering of the eyelids is known as blepharospasm. Fasciculations are often an intermittent problem, especially appearing at times of undue fatigue, or following undue muscular activity.

SYMPTOMATIC RELIEF OF MUSCULAR SYMPTOMS

There is no medical solution to muscular fatigue and weakness – the cardinal symptom of M.E. Patients have to learn to perform within their individual limitations by balancing exercise with adequate periods of rest. My practical approach to exercise and rest is dealt with in further detail on pages 140–6.

Muscle pain tends to respond rather badly to conventional mild analgesics that can be bought over the counter at the pharmacy. Aspirin remains an excellent anti-inflammatory drug if you have no problems with side-effects – so do use it if it helps. An alternative is to use one of the new non-steroidal anti-inflammatory drugs (NSAIDs), which can be prescribed by the doctor. One drug, ibuprofen (Brufen), can be purchased without prescription. These NSAIDs have to be used with caution as some M.E. sufferers seem to be unduly sensitive. They can cause stomach ulceration and bleeding. More worrying is recent research which suggests that long-term use can result in thinning of the bones. These drugs are now available as ointments – something which may be worth a try.

There are more potent pain killers available on prescription, but once again they tend to provide only limited relief. The risk is that you become dependent on them, so most doctors are quite rightly reluctant to prescribe them continually without very good reason.

Other aids are locally applied aspirin-like cream (triethanolamine salicylate – TEAS), which has recently been used with some success in America, but is not yet available in the U.K., and the spray-on pain relief aerosols, which tend to provide only a very short period of relief, and are therefore of little value.

Simple self-help measures can be quite effective:

- Use locally applied heat from a hot-water bottle, or lie in a warm bath.
- Massage the affected area using an embrocation from the pharmacy, such as Deep Heat; some patients even find horse linament beneficial.

If conventional approaches do not seem to help, it might be worth trying acupuncture or seeing an osteopath, particularly if the pain is in the back – see pages 154–5 and 173–4. However, if pain is a continuous and disabling part of your illness, unrelieved by any of the above, your doctor does have the option of referring you to a pain relief clinic. Most large district general hospitals now have such clinics, often run by the anaesthetists, but with help from other specialists as well – and sometimes these offer alternative approaches like acupuncture, counselling, and new ideas such as transcutaneous electrical stimulation. This involves applying small electrodes on to the skin, directly over a site of chronic pain. A small pulsed current is passed, which is thought to stimulate the production of endorphins, the body's natural pain killers. Details of how to find a pain relief clinic can be found on page 209.

RESEARCH INTO MUSCLE ABNORMALITIES IN M.E. PATIENTS

One of the objects of research into M.E. has been to clearly demonstrate that there are abnormalities in patients' muscles – and that the problem is in the muscle and not in the mind.

Muscle weakness can have many different causes, depending on which part of the nervous system, or the muscle itself, is not functioning properly. Messages to move or contract a particular muscle group originate in the brain, from where they pass down the spinal cord to the peripheral nerves, which then control the individual muscles. Between the end of the nerve and the start of the muscle fibre is a very important gap, known as the neuro-muscular junction. The message to contract the muscle is conducted across the gap by chemicals known as neurotransmitters. When the message reaches its destination, the muscle fibre contracts and so the arm or leg moves. Muscle weakness can therefore originate anywhere along this pathway.

Patients with spinal cord injuries are obviously unable to pass on the messages below the site of the damage, and so may be unable to move both arms and legs. In conditions like multiple sclerosis it is the peripheral nerves that are at fault, and in myasthenia gravis the weakness results from abnormalities in the chemical transmission of the messages across the junction. M.E. patients are often referred to neurologists because of their muscle weakness, and unless the neurologist is informed about M.E. a mistaken diagnosis may be made.

To go about detecting the site of possible muscle damage (myopathy) in M.E. patients, researchers have made use of three investigative techniques: electromyograms, muscle biopsies and nuclear magnetic resonance (N.M.R.).

Electromyograms (EMGs) These give the doctor a picture of how the patient's muscle fibres are responding to the electrical stimuli passing down the nerve fibres telling them to contract. Ordinary EMGs had already shown some minor abnormalities in the early Royal Free cases, but this information was of limited value.

Now, using a highly sophisticated form of this technique – known as single fibre electromyograms – neurophysiologists in Glasgow have found that most of the M.E. group tested had a very characteristic abnormality, which they referred to as 'abnormal jitter'. This abnormal jitter in the fibres suggested that there was a disturbance in the way the messages were being conducted along the muscle fibres, possibly as a result of damage to the surrounding membrane.

Muscle biopsies The second procedure was to take a small sliver of muscle (a biopsy) from the patient's leg using local anaesthetic, and then to examine it under the microscope for any abnormalities.

I was one of the patients under the first series of investigations in Glasgow, and so I had the interesting experience of watching the pathologist take the biopsy by making a two-inch incision in the skin just above my knee to reveal the muscle fibres, and then, just like cutting a piece of smoked salmon, removing a minute piece. The biopsies revealed several interesting abnormalities, but not every patient had identical changes.

The muscles are divided into two different groups of fibres. Type One fibres are said to be fatigue-resistant, and are thus able to withstand prolonged contraction, such as standing up for long periods. Type Two fibres are more concerned with fine movements, such as performing delicate tasks with the fingers or moving the eyes.

In many of the M.E. patients tested in Glasgow the normal ratio of the fibres was altered, showing an increase of Type Two fibres – those which are least likely to withstand prolonged fatigue, and this of course fits in with the type of muscular symptoms that M.E. patients complain of.

Under the microscope further changes were observed which suggested there had been damage in the muscle caused by the initial viral infection. Many of the patients had patchy areas of dead fibres (necrotic tissue), but there were no signs of any persisting inflammation.

Under very high-powered microscopes – electron microscopes – further changes became apparent. Electron microscopes make it possible to look at the individual structures within the muscle cells. One very important such structure is known as the mitochondria, or 'the power house of the cell' – it is here that energy is created within the muscle cell. In some of the M.E. patients tested, the mitochondria were abnormally increased in number and not situated in their usual sites, instead being found around the periphery of the cells. In addition, there were strange tubular inclusions, whose significance still remains uncertain.

Lastly, the research involved histochemical analysis, in which the cells were stained to assess the concentration of various enzymes within. Here the interesting discovery was made that some patients seemed to have reduced amounts of certain key enzymes concerned with mitochondrial function. In other words, here was supportive evidence for abnormal energy production.

Nuclear magnetic resonance The last, and probably most important part of the research into what was going wrong in the muscles involved co-operation with research workers in Oxford. Here, Professor George Radda was looking at various muscular diseases using a relatively new process called nuclear magnetic resonance (N.M.R.). This is a non-invasive procedure whereby the patient is placed in a giant cylindrical magnet through which the chemical reactions taking place in the muscle cells can be followed by computer. Dr Melvin Ramsay of the Royal Free asked if I could be the first M.E. patient to be investigated by this new technique, to see if there were any identifiable abnormalities in the way my muscles were producing their energy. I duly visited Oxford and the results confirmed that there was a unique biochemical defect in the way energy was being produced.

To understand the results of this experiment it is necessary to know how energy is produced in the muscle cells. Energy comes from carbohydrates in food, which are broken down by the digestive process and stored as glycogen in the muscle cells. Glycogen is the fuel which is burned up by exercise and, by a process known as glycolysis, converted into energy. For glycolysis to take place, two essential ingredients must be present. These are oxygen, brought to the muscles by the red blood cells, and enzymes, produced on site in the muscle cell, which act as catalysts in the burning process. When oxygen and enzymes are present in the right quantities, glycolysis takes place and energy is produced. This is known as aerobic metabolism. However, when oxygen is lacking, the result is anaerobic metabolism, in which excessive amounts of lactic acid are produced instead of energy.

Any normal human will produce some lactic acid as the result of muscular exercise, but when I was investigated with N.M.R. during exercise, there was a rapid and excessive production of lactic acid, indicating a significant abnormality in the way energy was being produced and consistent with the muscle fatigue I was experiencing.

N.M.R. investigations are costly, very time-consuming, and only available in one U.K. centre. They cannot be considered part of the routine investigation for anyone suspected of having M.E. As part of this research project a few other M.E. patients have also been assessed, with some, but not all showing similar changes.

Looking at another aspect of muscle abnormality in M.E. is Professor Timothy Peters, at London's Northwick Park Hospital, who is concentrating on the possibility that the virus may be using its own genetic code to switch off essential processes of protein synthesis and repair which the muscle cell must carry out in order to function properly. His initial findings, with the aid of muscle biopsies, suggest that M.E. patients are not able to produce new muscle proteins effectively, which must have important implications for all aspects of muscle cell activity. This looks like being important evidence to show that M.E. patients have a problem in their muscles, and not in their minds. Their fatigue is organic, not psychological.

It is not yet possible to tell how all these abnormalities fit together, and which could in the future be used as a basis for some form of treatment. There may be membrane damage resulting from the immune response; there could be a lack of oxygen getting through to the cells; and the virus actually inside the cell might be switching off the genetic codes, so that the cell is unable to carry out its normal functions.

Research into this vital part of the equation is moving forward very quickly – hopefully we should soon have some answers.

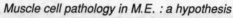

Muscle cell pathology in M.E. : a hypothesis

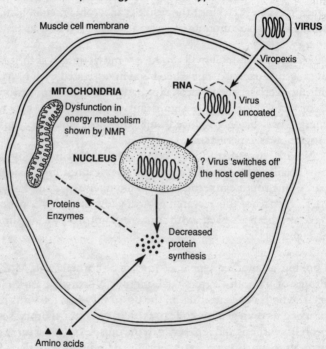

HOW M.E. AFFECTS THE BRAIN

Brain fatigue and malfunction – what doctors refer to as the encephalitic features of M.E. – are invariably a major part of the illness, but just like muscle fatigue, they tend to fluctuate in severity according to exertion. For many patients the day their brains stopped functioning properly is the most distressing feature of M.E., and for those whose employment depends on mental abilities the results can be devastating.

Mental exertion from academic work, reading, attending meetings and any other kind of activity requiring a high degree of intellectual concentration soon causes a rapid deterioration in brain functioning, and patients describe how a cloud descends over the brain as their attention span rapidly shortens. Interestingly, excess physical activity will also cause intellectual fatigue, so at the end of say a walk or a spell in the garden it is not only the muscles that are not functioning – it is the brain as well.

The two commonest symptoms as brain function deteriorates are loss of concentration and loss of recent memory. Recent memory refers to any information that has entered the brain via ears or eyes within the past few minutes or hours. Longer-term memory loss for events in the past is not usually a problem, although a few sufferers do notice difficulties here. Inability to keep one's mind operating and correctly processing and storing incoming information makes mental activity possible for only short periods – few M.E. sufferers can carry on with a demanding mental task for more than half an hour; for most the period is much shorter. Even the plot of *Dallas* may become impossible to follow after the first thirty minutes! Once ability to concentrate has deteriorated patients (or their friends) may notice that they are using inappropriate or opposite words without realising it (e.g. saying 'hot' when they mean 'cold'), or are completely unable to remember a familiar word or name – what doctors call anomia.

The ability to perform previously learned and familiar procedures – even knotting a tie or doing up one's shoelaces – may become temporarily impossible during an episode of brain malfunction. Rest then restores the energy levels and relatively normal function returns. Clumsiness, especially when undertaking fine tasks like threading a needle, is very common, and many patients also experience difficulties in co-ordinating their legs on stairs, or coming off moving escalators – if they dare get on them in the first place! Handwriting often deteriorates in the course of writing a long letter – if the brain can supply the necessary information.

Whichever parts of the brain are involved in M.E., there certainly does not seem to be any dementing process, with a gradual progressive deterioration of mental abilities over the course of the illness. The features of intellectual malfunction characteristically tend to fluctuate in severity – the patient's mental functioning may be perfectly normal for a short period of time, and then deteriorate rapidly, usually after a burst of mental or physical activity.

This phenomenon strongly suggests that just as the muscle runs out of energy during exercise, so the brain does the same thing. Few people realise that for the brain to function effectively, it requires large amounts of energy, just like the muscles. Lack of energy to vital centres is probably only part of the explanation. If the virus is persisting and possibly entering the brain, the reason why different patients seem to have different problems with aspects of brain function may be that the virus affects only certain parts of each patient's brain. If it enters the temporal lobes, the patient will have particular difficulties with memory; if it enters the frontal lobes, there will be problems with reasoning and thought processes, or emotional symptoms.

Other theories are also quite feasible – it has been suggested that there may be a depletion of the chemical neurotransmitters, vital conductors of messages between the millions of nerve cells. This suggestion has also been put forward as a chemical cause for some types of depressive illness, as well as the brain malfunction seen in other neurological diseases. Then there is the theory that the persisting virus may be stimulating excess production of interferon, which could also cause neurological and emotional symptoms as seen in M.E. Hopefully the answers will appear before long.

As patients do not die from M.E., brain tissue is very rarely available for examination under the microscope to help follow up these theories. We have to rely on current investigative procedures to suggest where abnormalities in function may be occurring. The normal test for electrical activity in the brain is the electroencephalogram (EEG), where electrodes are placed on the patient's scalp and brainwave activity is recorded. These EEG recordings have not however provided any revealing findings as to exactly where things are going wrong in the brain.

Recently in the United States some patients have been having nuclear magnetic resonance scans of brain tissue, and these have shown some pin-point abnormalities. In one patient the changes were reported as coming and going as the symptoms fluctuated. One other form of brain scan – known as a PET scan – can look at the way the brain takes up glucose, and this type of procedure may in future be of help in examining how M.E. patients use energy for mental functioning. Lastly there are the clinical psychologists, who by testing various mental skills, can to some extent show which parts of the brain are not functioning properly, and it is now planned to look at some M.E. patients using their techniques.

Whatever and wherever is the cause of brain malfunction in M.E. patients, it remains a persisting and extremely disabling part of the illness. A few patients find their brain function improves but their muscle symptoms do not, or vice versa, but for many frequent mental incapacity brings sheer despair.

There is no drug treatment to help this aspect of M.E. Drugs used to increase blood flow to the brain are not appropriate, and antidepressant medication will not help loss of concentration or memory unless the sufferer is truly depressed as well. All one can say is that the brain needs to be fed like the rest of the body, so the M.E. patient should take particular care to eat regular nutritious meals. Recent experiments at the University of Virginia have shown that failing mental ability in the elderly can be improved by taking a drink with 50 gm glucose added – a finding that might be worth trying on M.E. patients.

Where a patient is having severe difficulties with mental functioning it may be worth asking to be referred to a clinical psychologist for an opinion and advice. These psychologists are often attached to neurological departments in hospitals or centres specialising in rehabilitation of stroke or head injury patients.

On a purely practical level, I personally find that when my brain is not functioning, there is absolutely no point in trying to press on. The best policy is to try and completely switch off – mentally and physically – for at least an hour. I go and lie down in a quiet room, completely relaxed, and find that this approach can mostly be quite successful in effecting a return to normal.

Unfortunately, on some days this method does not work, and then I have to accept that my brain just will not function effectively that day, and defer any attempts at mental activity for twenty-four hours.

HOW M.E. AFFECTS THE NERVES

The human nervous system consists of millions of individual nerve cells, which store and pass on information and instructions rather like a computer. The various control centres for all this nervous activity are situated in different parts of the brain. From here the messages pass down the spinal cord and then out via the numerous tiny nerves to muscles, blood vessels and the body organs which are under nervous control. One particularly important part of the nervous system affected by M.E. are the autonomic nerves.

THE AUTONOMIC NERVOUS SYSTEM

This consists of two complementary sets of nerves, known as the sympathetic and parasympathetic fibres, which both pass to the part of the body they are controlling, but have opposing functions. For example, the sympathetic nerves to the heart will speed up its rate, whereas the parasympathetic fibres will slow down the rate. These nerves are again controlled by 'higher centres' in the brain, particularly in the brain stem.

These nerves are called autonomic, because unlike the nerves which control muscle movements, we don't have much voluntary control over their actions. If we get very worried about something this will trigger activity in the sympathetic nerves and speed up the pulse rate quite automatically, but there's no way we can cancel out this automatic overactivity.

The autonomic nerves try to maintain a 'status quo' in the body, and exert control over a wide range of body functions. They pass to the heart, the intestines, and the bladder where they control the emptying functions. They also have a very important role in body temperature control.

TEMPERATURE CONTROL

One particularly important autonomic control centre in the brain is known as the hypothalamus, and it's from here that the body is programmed to maintain its constant internal temperature. It acts as an 'internal thermostat'.

M.E. patients invariably have various difficulties with their body temperature control, being abnormally sensitive to any extreme of temperature, be it a hot bath or climatic heat or cold. Patients often feel cold and shivery, and may even want to wrap up when the external temperature is quite warm. It's not unusual to record body temperatures with a thermometer constantly a degree or so below normal. One strange aspect of this, which I experience as an M.E. sufferer, is that whenever I succumb to an infection I rarely have a raised temperature, but just feel cold and shivery, and so take to bed with a jersey and hot-water bottle.

One of the normal body mechanisms for losing heat is to sweat, and profuse night sweats (just like those some women experience during their menopause) are quite a common feature. Sweating may also be noticed by some patients when they try to 'push on' – mentally or physically – beyond their limitations.

Unfortunately, there's no effective medical therapy for these problems with temperature regulation apart from avoiding, wherever possible, situations where they might occur. This is particularly appropriate if you go on holiday to hot climates and stay out too long in the sun, thinking it's bound to be beneficial.

THE HEART AND BLOOD VESSELS

M.E., through dysfunction of the nervous system, can also affect the heart and the small blood vessels. Overactivity in the sympathetic nervous system can cause a sudden increase in the pulse rate (a tachycardia) and this may be accompanied by the frightening sensation of actually feeling the heart beating inside the chest – palpitations. These palpitations will be exacerbated if the sufferer is also feeling anxious. If you experience either rapid pulse rates or palpitations, it's very important to avoid anything else which can overstimulate these nerves, including coffee, alcohol, and even the contents of some cold cures and nasal sprays. If in doubt do ask your pharmacist.

There are drugs available, known as beta-blockers, which can dampen down this overactivity and help to control symptoms, and where palpitations are particularly bothersome such treatment may be worth trying. Before using these drugs your doctor may wish to check the heart rhythm using an electrocardiogram (ECG), just to make sure that there's no other problem with the heart itself. One of the disadvantages of using beta-blockers is that like all drugs they have side-effects, some of which can be similar to the symptoms already caused by M.E.

The sympathetic nerves also alter the size of the tiny blood vessels which supply blood to the hands and feet. The ghastly facial pallor which may be noticed before a patient feels grossly fatigued may be part of this malfunction, if blood supply to the skin is reduced. Cold hands and feet are a common accompaniment to M.E., and are often brought on by cold weather, when these tiny blood vessels seem to be unduly sensitive and clamp down. Inhalation of cigarette smoke can also worsen the problem. Beta-blockers can exacerbate these symptoms, as well as the feelings of fatigue. The exact drug needs to be chosen with care, and this usually means using one whose effects are primarily on the nerves to the heart (a cardioselective one), and at a low enough dose to be both effective, and hopefully free from side-effects.

The most effective way of dealing with the problems of cold hands and feet is by the following simple practical advice:

- Don't smoke cigarettes, and avoid other people's smoke.
- Wear adequate woolly clothing (i.e. several layers) when going outside in cold weather.
- Keep at least one area of the house constantly warm during the day in cold weather.
- Don't warm up cold hands by putting them straight on to a hot radiator – they *must* be rewarmed gradually.

If cold hands and feet are causing a lot of difficulties, especially outdoors in winter, it may be worth taking more radical measures, and purchasing some battery-heated shoes and gloves. The Raynaud's Association Trust (address on page 211) deals specifically with this condition, and can give further practical advice and help.

Although many patients experience palpitations and rapid pulse rates from time to time, this doesn't mean that the heart has become affected by the illness. The most likely reason is an overactivity of the sympathetic nerves which are telling it to start beating faster.

However, there are a few patients with M.E. who do have associated heart disease, because, as mentioned earlier, the enteroviruses can affect both the heart muscle (the myocardium = myocarditis) or the heart lining (the pericardium = pericarditis). In these cases the patient is often quite seriously ill at the beginning, due to the effects on the heart, and may have to be admitted to hospital. In many cases this heart involvement will completely settle down, but in a few these problems will continue. Previously doctors explained these patients' fatigue as being the result of poor output of blood from the damaged heart tissues. Although this is an important factor, it's now recognised that some of these 'heart patients' do have M.E. as well.

I must stress that this direct involvement of the heart is very unusual, but it can occur. If you are having persistent chest pains and palpitations your doctor will probably want to do some tests (e.g. an electrocardiogram to trace the heart rhythm), just to be sure there's nothing more serious going wrong.

FEELING FAINT OR FAINTING

One further important function of the autonomic nerves is that of controlling our blood pressure by their effect on the size of the larger blood vessels. If these vessels are too dilated, then the pressure in the system falls, not enough blood reaches the brain, and we either feel faint or actually faint. When we move from lying or sitting to a standing position these vessels should contract to keep blood flowing to the brain, but some M.E. sufferers find they feel faint on suddenly standing up, and this is what doctors call postural hypotension – a fall in blood pressure on standing.

Postural hypotension probably isn't the only reason why some M.E. patients feel faint at times. In some of the earlier outbreaks of M.E., a few patients were found to have very low blood sugars (hypoglycaemia) and were even admitted to hospital unconscious because of this. Another factor may be related to any drugs being taken. Antidepressant drugs can lower blood pressure as a side-effect, as can alcohol, and excessive heat.

If this symptom seems to be a particular problem it's worth asking your doctor to check your blood pressure, to see if it does fall significantly when you change from lying to standing.

Whatever the cause, there are measures *you* can take:

- If postural hypotension is the problem, be very careful about how you move from lying to standing. Learn to exercise your stomach muscles by pulling them in several times before changing position – this helps to raise the blood pressure – and get up slowly.
- If you're getting hypoglycaemic take regular meals, and carry a supply of glucose tablets to take if necessary.

If the problem is very troublesome, there are drugs which can be prescribed, but they require very careful consideration, and are outside the scope of this book.

UNSTEADINESS AND DIZZINESS

The almost constant unsteadiness reported by many patients is a further example of the way M.E. is probably affecting parts of the nervous system responsible for balance. These symptoms may result in M.E. sufferers being referred for repeated visits to ENT (ear, nose and throat) doctors, who like their colleagues can't find anything wrong. Again, the routine tests may be normal, and the type of investigations which show up abnormalities in this part of the nervous system may only be available in specialised centres.

Unsteadiness and dizziness is a very common medical problem, with a large number of possible causes, including anxiety, which may then be queried as the underlying problem. There are a large number of drugs designed to help, but in the case of M.E. their value seems very limited, and I do not know of many patients who have benefited.

Neurologists interested in the practical difficulties associated with dizziness (vertigo) have devised a series of exercises designed to improve balance, but again I haven't found them to be of any benefit.

BLADDER DYSFUNCTION

This can form an additional part to the other disturbances occurring in M.E. Some of the autonomic nerves help to contract the muscles of the bladder wall and cause emptying, whereas others help to keep the bladder exit sphincter closed till the body wishes to pass urine.

Symptoms such as frequently wanting to pass urine, getting up in the night to pass urine or the feeling of having an 'irritable bladder' seem fairly common in both men and women with M.E.

Poor muscle control may be the reason some men have a poor urinary stream and dribble at the end. Occasionally, when a man gets up in the middle of the night to pass urine he will faint in the process, again due to the wrong messages in these nerves.

In women there may be weakness of the pelvic floor muscles and this may produce what's known as stress incontinence. Here sudden abdominal pressure from coughing, straining or exercise can suddenly produce an embarrassing leak of urine, as the pelvic muscles fail to contract properly around the urethra. If this is happening, a properly taught course of pelvic floor exercises will probably help. Also, a recently researched method is now being taught which involves the patient inserting cones of varying sizes into the vagina for short periods each day, and the effort of keeping the cones in place specifically strengthens the weak pelvic muscles.

If you do want to pass urine frequently, your doctor will probably want to exclude any infection by sending a specimen to the laboratory, but this would usually be recommended when some pain is present as well (dysuria). If no infection is present then the reason may well be to do with the nervous control of bladder function. The doctor may also decide to carry out a full investigation of the whole urinary tract from kidneys to bladder, by doing an IVP test (intravenous pyelogram), but with M.E.

sufferers this is very unlikely to show up any abnormality specific to M.E.

More sophisticated techniques are now available in specialised urological units to accurately assess the nerve–muscle control of bladder function. It would be interesting to now examine some M.E. patients who have bladder problems using these techniques to try and get a better idea of what's going wrong in this aspect of M.E.

If bladder symptoms such as frequency are becoming very incapacitating there are some drugs which may be of help, but again would only be prescribed after careful consideration.

DISTURBANCES INVOLVING SENSORY NERVES

One last part of the nervous system which seems to be affected in some patients are the sensory nerves, which carry information on sensation, pain, pressure and temperature change back to the brain. If there are problems here, such symptoms as numbness (hypoaesthesiae), 'pins and needles' (paraesthesiae) or sometimes an increased awareness of sensation (hyperaesthesiae) can occur.

I'd had M.E. for about five years before ever experiencing any of these changes. Then one very cold November day I'd been out walking my dog, and on returning home I noticed that my right foot had started to feel cold and numb. Over the following few days I also started to develop pins and needles in my fingers. These symptoms continued intermittently all through the winter till spring arrived, and now they return each year, in varying degrees of severity according to how cold the weather is.

Many other M.E. sufferers also notice that these sensory changes tend to come and go, and particularly affect the hands and feet, but are not necessarily related to the cold. A few patients also notice altered sensations on their tongues and inside their mouths.

There are no obvious medical solutions to these abnormal sensations. They can have many other different causes, some of them treatable, and it's important, that if such symptoms come on after M.E. has been present for some time, the doctor carries out some investigations to exclude all other possibilities. Various vitamin B supplements are often prescribed by doctors for these sensory symptoms, but their value in M.E. is doubtful unless a specific deficiency can be demonstrated.

4. Secondary Problems

The cardinal symptoms of M.E., discussed in the previous chapter, are joined in some patients as the disease progresses by secondary symptoms affecting other parts of the body.

Although you may have cleared the first hurdle and got your doctor to accept that M.E. really does exist – causing muscle fatigue and brain malfunction – you may once again be facing an uphill struggle persuading him or her that these seemingly unrelated problems are also part of the disease process, and aren't due to the fact that you've now become depressed because you've got M.E. Many members of the medical profession have forgotten most of what they learnt about enteroviruses back at medical school, and just aren't aware of the diverse range of body tissues that they can affect. However, both doctors and patients should remember that it is unwise simply to blame the development of any new symptom on M.E. – there may be a completely unrelated problem which requires investigation and specific treatment.

THE EARS AND HEARING PROBLEMS

M.E. patients quite frequently remark on three particular problems connected with hearing:

- The presence of abnormal noises in the ear – tinnitus. These sounds can be high-pitched whistling or hissing, and particularly occur at times of stress or undue fatigue.
- Being unable to cope with constant chatter in a room full of people, or a lot of loud noise (hyperacusis). Hyperacusis may alternate with periods of deafness or normal hearing.
- Pain in or around the ear.

Normally sound is transmitted in waves through the various components of the outer and middle ear to a structure called the cochlea. This is a fluid-filled chamber with thousands of tiny hair cells lining its walls. Sound vibrations pass through it moving the tiny hairs, and thus the message is transformed into a nerve impulse, which passes along the auditory nerve (or nerve of hearing) to the brain, where it is decoded. It seems that in M.E. patients the ability of the auditory nerve to conduct sound waves suffers from interference – rather like a faulty telephone wire.

Tinnitus is an extremely distressing accompaniment to M.E. – especially if present for much of the time, which makes any form of concentration even more difficult. There is no effective drug treatment for tinnitus, although some doctors will prescribe tranquillisers where stress is a factor, but these drugs are not a long-term solution. Fortunately, in many cases, the symptom is intermittent, and in my personal experience it can disappear altogether for quite long periods of time.

If tinnitus is persistent and troublesome then an ENT (ear, nose and throat) surgeon may recommend trying what is known as a 'masking device'. This acts rather like a hearing aid, and masks the unpleasant noise with a pleasant background sound. An alternative do-it-yourself method for masking tinnitus is using a personal stereo to play soothing music. The Tinnitus Association (see page 212) can provide further information and practical advice if necessary.

EYES AND VISUAL DISTURBANCES

M.E. is capable of causing several visual disturbances:

Blurring of vision (defective accommodation) This is very common, especially after prolonged periods of watching television or reading print in a newspaper or book. The words become increasingly difficult to focus on and may start to appear double (double vision = diplopia). The cause is probably related to the fact that correct focusing of the eye is controlled by tiny muscles – ciliary muscles – and just like other muscles in M.E. patients they are prone to fatigue after prolonged use.

Some patients make repeated visits to the optician to try and get the problem sorted out. The optician, not surprisingly, finds nothing wrong. So, for M.E. patients, it is important not to visit your optician on an 'off day', feeling exhausted, with your vision worse than usual.

Photophobia – dislike of bright lights – is also quite common, and this may stem from increased sensitivity to light in the brain. If patients cannot avoid shops, working areas, etc., where there are very bright lights, they should try wearing dark glasses when necessary.

Pain in and around the eyes can be quite severe, and become localised behind one eye (retro-orbital pain). The doctor may query a diagnosis of migraine, but the pain is not usually associated with the sickness or visual disturbances seen in migraine. This type of eye pain does not tend to respond well to analgesics, and often all you can do is rest quietly until it goes away.

GASTRIC UPSETS AND PROBLEMS RELATED TO EATING

M.E. patients seem to have a lot of problems with their digestion and bowels, and some people can get unduly worried about such symptoms, which is only likely to make them worse. So, if you have gastric problems, do discuss them with your doctor, get any tests done that seem appropriate to rule out any other causes, and try some of the drugs available to help relieve the symptoms.

In a few patients food sensitivity or allergy may be a problem, but please do not embark on any drastic dietary alterations without expert supervision.

M.E. seems capable of causing a wide variety of digestive problems, with a large number of patients having persisting or fluctuating symptoms, including nausea, vague colicky stomach pains, bloating, and alterations in bowel habit, which can veer towards diarrhoea or constipation. Vomiting, progressive weight loss or blood in the motions should *not* be ascribed to M.E., and a search must be made for an alternative explanation.

Some patients do lose some weight in the early stages of the illness and then experience great difficulty in putting it on again later, no matter how hard they try. It has also been observed that children with M.E. seem to have considerable difficulty putting on weight during their illness.

Trying to establish the reason for these symptoms so that a treatment can be devised is not easy, but a number of explanations have been put forward. The whole gastrointestinal tract consists of a long hosepipe-like tube which starts at the oesophagus. From here, food enters the stomach where digestion takes place, then it continues its journey through many feet of intestines where nutrients are absorbed and waste products excreted. The lining of the intestine is made up of cells which form a membrane called the mucosa. Surrounding the mucosa are layers of muscle fibres, whose function is to rhythmically contract in a wave-like manner to propel the food and waste products along. Like any other muscle this is under nervous control, and may therefore be affected by the M.E. virus.

Where there is a combination of colicky stomach pain, bloating or wind, and alteration in normal bowel habit, the explanation may be what doctors term the 'irritable bowel syndrome'. This seems to be a common problem not only in M.E.; it has been estimated that about 15 per cent of all adults suffer from irritable bowel.

One suggested cause for irritable bowel is an overactivity of the nerves controlling the propulsive movements of the muscle in the bowel wall, and as these movements become unco-ordinated muscle spasm and pain result. It has been shown in experiments that if a balloon is introduced into the intestine, and the pressure inside it is increased, the characteristic colicky pain can be reproduced. As a result of this abnormal or increased propulsion of bowel contents there may also be diarrhoea. It has been suggested that gastric infections may initiate the development of irritable bowel, and it is not unknown for this condition to develop after a nasty stomach upset caught abroad on holiday.

Intolerance of or abnormal sensitivity to certain foods may also be a factor in irritable bowel.

Whatever causes irritable bowel in the first place the symptoms will inevitably be exacerbated by any associated anxiety about the condition, so it is worth emphasising that it has no serious consequences, cannot lead to cancer, and frequently resolves or improves in the course of time. The way the medical profession treats irritable bowel is by trying to alleviate the individual symptoms. The colicky pain may be helped by drugs that have a direct relaxing effect on the muscle. Colofac is one such drug, but it requires a prescription from your doctor. A course of capsules containing peppermint oil (Colpermin, available over the counter) is an alternative that may be worth trying. This also relaxes the intestinal muscles to help with colic and bloating, though some patients find it causes side-effects including gastric irritation and heartburn.

The most popular method of managing irritable bowel symptoms is an increase in dietary fibre. This means ensuring that the diet is rich in fruit, vegetables and wholemeal bread, or even adding bran directly on to food, such as the morning breakfast cereal. This sort of dietary change has to be introduced gradually (especially if you are going to try added bran), as a drastic change in diet may exacerbate symptoms, and increased fibre does not suit all patients. In a few patients, where nerve-muscle control seems to be at fault, increasing fibre can lead to more pain and bloating. In this case one of the now unfashionable stimulant laxatives (e.g. Senna) may be helpful.

Wind and bloating or flatulence can often be helped by a preparation containing Dimethicone, which helps to make the wind bubbles in the stomach coalesce. When constipation is the predominant symptom, it may help to use a laxative that increases the bulk contents of the stools, such as Fybogel or Isogel. These drugs help the stool to retain water, so expanding the size, and thus increasing the motility.

If diarrhoea accompanies the pain, then management is rather different. The diarrhoea of irritable bowel is not usually like that of true infective diarrhoea – it has the consistency of toothpaste, and may alternate with normal stools, or constipated pellet-like motions. In a phase of diarrhoea, a prescribed anti-diarrhoeal drug such as codeine phosphate or loperamide (Imodium) may be useful. If you have persisting watery diarrhoea a stool sample should be sent to the local laboratory to check for infection, although enteroviral infection cannot be detected by standard techniques. Your doctor may also wish to arrange further hospital investigations including a sigmoidoscopy (a look inside the lower bowel using a long flexible tube) or barium examination, just to make sure there is nothing more serious going on.

Blood in the motions is *not* part of irritable bowel (or M.E.); if this occurs you *must* go to your doctor – it may simply be piles, but it could indicate something more significant.

Abnormal nerve-muscle control of the bowel wall may be only part of the explanation for the diverse range of gastric upsets seen in M.E. patients. We now know from the research work at St Mary's Hospital, London, that many M.E. patients have a persisting enteroviral infection in the gut, and this reservoir of infection may be inflaming the lining mucosa and surrounding muscle to produce food sensitivities, intolerance or allergy. If this is the problem, one possible approach is to try an exclusion diet, which usually involves cutting out suspect foods – such as coffee, cereals, dairy produce – one by one over longish periods until the culprit or culprits have been isolated. A more drastic method is to restrict the diet to spring water, one source of protein (e.g. chicken) and one carbohydrate (e.g. potatoes), plus some vitamins, for seven days to see if there is any improvement. Then, groups of foods can be gradually reintroduced to see if they provoke symptoms.

This sort of dietary manipulation should be carried out only with careful thought and with the help of an interested doctor or dietician – after all, M.E. sufferers have enough restrictions imposed on their lives already without restricting their food intake.

WEIGHT GAIN AND M.E.

Although neither significant nor progressive weight loss is a part of M.E., some patients do experience the opposite problem and find that their weight is gradually increasing. The new relatively inactive lifestyle imposed by M.E. obviously decreases the body's energy requirements quite substantially, so some patients may find that they have to cut down their calories accordingly. This should be done by reducing the sugar and fat content in the normal diet, not by any dramatic starvation-type diets involving a very low calorie intake.

Weight gain can occasionally be associated with a hormonal problem, and if underactivity of the thyroid gland is suspected your doctor will want to take some blood tests to check the thyroid function.

NAUSEA

Some patients experience intermittent feelings of nausea (sickness), though this is not usually associated with vomiting. Why this should be is not certain – there is an area in the brain, which if disturbed, can cause a feeling of sickness; nausea can also be associated with anxiety.

If necessary there is a variety of drugs that can help, but it is preferable not to take any on a long-term basis, especially those in the phenothiazine group (e.g. Stemetil), which can have side-effects on the nervous system. Two natural solutions reported as being effective are root ginger and acupressure. Acupressure is similar to acupuncture but involves pressure to a precise point on the wrist (the Neiguan point). This is achieved by an elasticated wrist band and a stud which presses on this acupressure site, about three fingers above the first wrist crease.

OESOPHAGEAL SPASM

Spasms in the oesophagus (throat) tend to come and go and may cause difficulty with swallowing. Such spasms may be related to those elsewhere in the gut which cause irritable bowel. Any continual difficulty with swallowing is a symptom you must see the doctor about, as it will require further investigation. If oesophageal spasm is the difficulty then there are drugs that can help, but you must take the advice of an experienced gastroenterologist.

PROCTALGIA FUGAX

This is the name given to a severe cramp-like pain in the anus. It often comes on suddenly, but may then last for up to half an hour or so before gradually starting to subside. Some relief may be obtained by going to the toilet, or having a warm bath, otherwise there is no effective treatment. Tranquillisers should be avoided if possible. The connection with M.E., as with oesophageal spasm, is muscular and nervous disturbance.

PRE-MENSTRUAL TENSION (PMT)

If you're unlucky enough to have both M.E. and the symptoms of pre-menstrual tension, the two conditions are going to interact and make each other seem worse. PMT symptoms characteristically start towards the latter part of the cycle from the time of ovulation, and then rapidly improve within a day or so of starting the period. There is a long list of symptoms, both mental and physical, associated with PMT, but among the commonest are irritability, depression, stomach bloating and breast enlargement or pain (mastalgia).

Popular self-help measures include taking Evening Primrose oil (Efamol) and vitamin B6 (Pyridoxine), in doses of 50–150 mgm daily, starting three days before the usual onset of symptoms and continuing until the period starts. There are reports of higher doses of vitamin B6 causing nervous inflammation, so use with care! Some patients gain benefit from the sort of relaxation techniques described on pages 76–7, along with a well-balanced diet – possibly avoiding coffee, chocolates, additives and sugar, but again advantages are not scientifically proven.

One theory as to the cause of PMT is hormonal imbalance, with a reduction in progesterone and an excess of oestrogen occurring at this time of the cycle. For this reason many gynaecologists prescribe extra progesterone. Where fluid retention and breast tenderness is the main problem a diuretic (water-losing drug) may help. If breast symptoms are very marked there are other drugs affecting the hormone levels that can be tried.

There is no simple solution to PMT; what suits one patient may not help another, so trying several different approaches may be necessary before relief is obtained. Further help and advice from National Association for Pre-Menstrual Syndrome (see page 208).

THE MENOPAUSE AND OSTEOPOROSIS

The menopause is the time of life when the ovaries start to decrease their production of the hormone oestrogen. The first sign may be an increasing irregularity in the pattern and blood loss of periods – though this should not automatically be ascribed to the menopause. Some women start to experience menopausal symptoms as early as forty, whereas others may be over fifty before anything changes. Many women go through the menopause with no problems at all, but in some the falling levels of oestrogen produce definite symptoms such as hot flushes, sweats, and aching joints. Vague emotional symptoms may also occur, including irritability and depression – just as with PMT.

The problem for any woman with M.E. who is approaching the menopause is that many of the symptoms overlap, particularly vasomotor instability (hot flushes, night sweats, palpitations), which is probably due to the autonomic nerve malfunction described on page 43. Consequently the two conditions will interact to exacerbate one another.

If there is any doubt as to whether the vasomotor symptoms are due to M.E. or to the menopause, the latter is the likely cause if there are associated changes in period pattern, with vaginal dryness and a rise in the hormone FSH, which can be measured by your doctor. Vaginal dryness may cause pain during sexual intercourse and this can be helped by increasing the lubrication with KY Jelly (from the pharmacy) or a locally applied oestrogen cream available on prescription.

Another problem related to the menopause is osteoporosis – loss of calcium and consequent thinning of bones – a natural ageing process, but one that accelerates in women going through the menopause because of the dramatic fall of oestrogen levels. Osteoporotic bones, especially in the wrist and hip, become fragile and susceptible to fracture.

Female M.E. sufferers of any age who are already thin and inactive (which also increases calcium loss), and who do not get outside in the sunlight to absorb vitamin D, are increasing their chances of developing osteoporosis, especially if they are also on a diet excluding milk and other dairy products – foods rich in calcium. Cigarette smoking is another contributory factor.

To try and minimise the risk of developing osteoporosis, any M.E. sufferer who is not taking adequate calcium in her diet should be taking some form of calcium supplement (e.g. Sandocal tablets, which can be made into a fizzy drink, or ordinary calcium tablets from the pharmacy), but *do not exceed* the recommended doses, as excess calcium can be harmful.

Hormone replacement therapy (HRT), now widely advocated by the medical profession, is something to be seriously considered by any M.E. sufferer entering the menopause, as it not only helps the vasomotor symptoms, but slows down the calcium loss caused by the falling oestrogen levels. In addition, it is believed to give increased protection against heart disease. HRT should be discussed with your doctor, and may be a viable option provided there are no medical contra-indications – e.g. heart disease, previous cancer of the breast or uterus.

THRUSH

Candida albicans, or thrush, is probably the commonest cause of vaginal discharge in women. For some, though, it is not just an occasional 'one-off' problem, but a recurring nuisance which never seems to go away.

The yeast candida often lives quite happily in our bodies without causing any problems. Then, from time to time, it gets out of control and multiplies to start causing definite symptoms. In the vagina this is a creamy discharge along with external soreness and irritation, but other parts of the body, particularly the skin and nails, can also be affected.

A variety of explanations have been put forward as to what 'tips the balance', and allows the yeast to start multiplying. These include courses of antibiotics, diabetes and immune-deficiency. Many gynaecologists now doubt that there is any link between thrush and taking the oral contraceptive pill. The fact that it is a latent organism prone to periodic reactivation has caused some doctors to link it with M.E., but in my personal view incidence of thrush is not much higher among M.E. patients than elsewhere in the population. I am dealing with it here for the benefit of those patients who do believe there is a link.

Treatment of an acute episode of thrush is usually very effective; it is preventing recurrence that causes the problem. Pessaries are the commonest prescribed treatment – these used to have to be inserted for a week or more, but now there are new types of pessary which are equally effective in a few days, or can even be taken in one 'megadose'. Some women prefer the anti-fungal creams, which can be prescribed along with an applicator, and are also very effective. Your male partner may also have the infection on his penis, and without any symptoms, so it is usually a good idea to get him to use some cream twice daily also.

Self-help measures can significantly reduce the chances of a recurrence:

- Avoid tight-fitting jeans, nylon pants and tights – in fact any clothing that helps to create a warm, moist environment in which the yeast thrives.
- Wipe your bottom away from your vagina as reinfection can come from the bowels.
- Do not 'traumatise' the vagina by using chemicals like bubble baths in the bath or vaginal douches; if you are dry during intercourse use some KY Jelly.

Some patients find the use of natural yogurt prepared with Lactobacillus helpful, although recent research from Sweden has questioned its value.

If you do keep getting recurrences of thrush your doctor may be willing to give you a further supply of medication, or a prescription, so you can start treatment yourself as soon as any symptoms recur.

If none of this seems to help then a prolonged course of anti-fungal treatment may be necessary.

PAIN IN THE JOINTS

In addition to the muscle pain (myalgia) which may accompany the fatigue in M.E., some patients also experience a variety of joint and bone pains. This kind of pain – arthralgia – is not usually as severe as the muscle pain, and is not associated with any permanent disruption to the joint, which can occur in purely rheumatic diseases.

If the joints are carefully examined by the doctor it is unusual to find any restriction in their range of movements and there are no changes seen with X-rays. For these reasons the cause may well be due to involvement of the supporting structures – muscles and tendons – which surround the joint. However, it is also recognised that a variety of viral infections can cause a temporary arthritis, with rubella being particularly common. And it has been suggested that viruses may persist inside cells known as chondrocytes, which produce the joint cartilage.

If you are experiencing joint pains, particularly if there is any associated swelling, a search should be made by your doctor to exclude one of the rheumatic diseases before ascribing this symptom to M.E.

Treatment of arthralgia is normally with one of the anti-inflammatory drugs, whichever seems to suit the individual patient best. Aspirin, taken four to six hourly, is still a very effective drug if it does not upset the stomach. If this is unsuitable one of the new anti-inflammatory drugs (NSAIDs) can be purchased (e.g. Brufen) or prescribed, but they do not suit all M.E. patients. Paracetamol is not a very effective drug for arthritic pain, and steroids should *definitely* be avoided.

One useful alternative approach is Evening Primrose Oil (Efamol), which has been shown in scientifically controlled trials to be as effective as conventional drugs in some patients. It is free from any side-effects.

DISORDERED SLEEP

The average 'normal' adult varies widely in his or her nightly sleep requirements. Some can manage perfectly well with only a few hours each night, whereas others must have their statutory ten hours or more.

One thing in common to all M.E. patients is their greatly increased sleep requirements (hypersomnia), and the frequent need to have a sleep or 'cat nap' half way through the day. Very few M.E. patients seem able to cope with being up and about for a full twelve-hour day without some sort of rest, unless they're going through an extremely good patch. Even after a full night's sleep an M.E. patient will still awake unrefreshed.

Normal human sleep is divided into two quite distinct components, each one occurring in alternating periods throughout the night. Dream sleep occurs for about a quarter of the total time asleep, coming on in bursts of gradually increasing length. During this dream sleep the body muscles relax and dreams occur. This type of sleep state is technically known as rapid eye movement (REM) sleep.

The other type of sleep – orthodox or non-REM sleep – occurs in rather longer periods between each period of dream sleep. During these periods you pass gradually from a light sleep into deep sleep and then re-enter your periods of dream sleep.

Control of sleep is thought to centre in the brain stem and hypothalamus. As has already been mentioned, disturbances in these areas are thought to be part of M.E., so this may explain why M.E. patients have such disordered sleep patterns. Whether M.E. patients have significant changes in the ratio of dream sleep and non-dream sleep is probably an area that warrants further research.

The pattern of sleep disturbance in M.E. is quite varied. Besides the common complaint of being 'tired all the time' and excessive sleep requirements generally, some patients may find themselves falling asleep at inappropriate times of the day, even before taking their afternoon nap! In a few unfortunate cases there is a complete reversal of the normal sleeping pattern, where the sufferer finds himself more alert at night and wanting to sleep during the day.

At night there are three types of disturbed sleep pattern commonly reported:

(1) Difficulty getting to sleep Although the sufferer may feel quite exhausted after a day's activities (or lack of) they still find that they can't get off to sleep, and sometimes this coincides with a rapid rise in mental activity as they lie in bed trying to start the night's sleep. These thoughts may be related to the things they planned and haven't managed to get done during the day, plans for the future or a range of miscellaneous unsolvable worries.

(2) Waking up once asleep This affects some M.E. patients and the cause can be associated with distressing physical symptoms preventing continued sleep, e.g. muscle aches and cramps, back pains, restless legs or jerking movements. These sort of physical symptoms may continually interrupt the sleep pattern throughout the night, making the sufferer feel even worse the next morning.

Night cramps in the calf muscles can affect anyone, and if

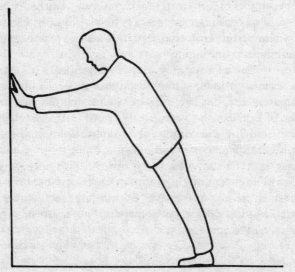

massage or local heat won't provide relief a simple stretching exercise can often be very effective in relieving the pain.

Stand and face the bedroom wall, with feet about three feet away from the skirting board. Then lean forward using hands and arms to act as support against the wall, making sure that the heels don't move off the ground. This will stretch the calf muscles: keep them stretched for about ten seconds, then relax for a while and repeat the exercise.

If cramp is occurring regularly try repeating these exercises three times a day as well.

A wide range of drugs have also been tried for treating night cramps (Quinine sulphate is frequently prescribed), but there's no general agreement as to their value.

Restless legs are another cause of restless nights, whereby sufferers complain of a variety of strange sensations, which seem to be more in the muscle than in the skin. (Doctors sometimes refer to this condition as Ekbom's Syndrome.) Tickling, pricking, burning or crawling feelings are frequently mentioned, and some patients also experience jerking movements in the legs. This strange activity is usually confined to the lower parts of the leg; the thigh and ankle areas are not usually affected.

The symptoms seem to gradually increase in intensity, till the only way of obtaining any relief is to get out of bed and walk around the room. Unfortunately, this may have to be repeated several times in one night.

Doctors don't know what causes 'restless legs'; it's certainly not confined to M.E. sufferers, and has also been linked with rheumatoid arthritis, iron deficiency anaemia, and an excessive intake of caffeine – so perhaps it's worth trying decaffeinated coffee. Sometimes warming (or cooling) the affected leg may help; other sufferers try exercises before going to sleep, but there doesn't seem to be any effective treatment which suits everyone.

As with night cramps, a variety of drugs have been tried, but the results are not impressive. Fortunately, for many people awoken by this strange phenomenon it's a transient problem which seems to come and go.

Vivid dreams, or even nightmares are also reported by some M.E. sufferers. These dreams are often described as being in vivid colours and involving various 'pressures' which seem to be worrying the patient, e.g. getting back to work again, or the frustrations of trying to achieve some other impossible task.

(3) Early morning wakening In this a third sleep disturbance reported in M.E., the sufferer wakes at, say, 4 or 5 a.m., and then has great difficulty in getting back to sleep again. This type of sleep disturbance can also be a very marked feature of depression, so it may point to the fact that an M.E. sufferer is becoming depressed, and needs professional help and treatment.

HELPING YOURSELF TO A BETTER NIGHT'S SLEEP

There are some useful tips which may help in getting a better night's sleep, without having to resort to a prescription for sleeping tablets.

- Try not to involve yourself in stimulating mental activity in the hour before you normally go to sleep. For example reading a small amount from a book can be very helpful in 'switching off'.
- If you don't feel relaxed last thing at night try the relaxation techniques described on pages 76–7, especially if you have any painful 'trouble spots'.
- Don't take any stimulants late in the evening such as tea, coffee or alcohol. A warm milky drink or a herbal tea is a much better alternative.
- If pain is waking you up in the night or preventing you getting to sleep try taking a mild pain killer before you retire.
- If you're not feeling too tired, sex is a very good way of sending people off to sleep!

HOW THE DOCTOR CAN HELP

Unfortunately this tends to be by prescribing some form of sleeping drug – hypnotic drugs. If poor sleep is associated with depression then one of the sedating antidepressant drugs mentioned later may be of help. However, many drugs have side-effects which include drowsiness, light headedness, confusion, and dizziness the following day. You can see why they're not a very good idea in M.E. when you're probably having these problems already, and why learning relaxation techniques is a much better alternative.

The use of any sleeping tablet must be restricted to only a short period of use. Dependence soon occurs and their value in promoting useful sleep slowly diminishes. Most M.E. patients have some form of long-term problem with sleep disturbances, and hypnotic drugs are not the answer.

It's important to remember that the commonest sleep problem in M.E. – that of requiring too much sleep – isn't something to fight against. This is your body's way of instructing you to rest and slow down, and it's also a very important healing mechanism, which allows the body to repair its damaged tissues and aid recovery. So don't feel guilty about having a short sleep in the afternoon, or going to bed early if you feel the need to. If your body says 'sleep' then this is what you really must do.

MIND AND BODY

'If you don't think that you're ever going to get better, then you probably never will.'

Taken literally, such a dramatic statement is not entirely applicable to something like M.E., but there's no doubt that there's more than a grain of truth in it. Attitude of mind – both positive and negative – is going to have a very significant effect on many aspects of M.E., as it can with many other similar conditions.

The primary effect may simply be on your 'coping mechanisms' – i.e. how you're able to deal with all the frustrations, anxieties and problems associated with M.E. It also seems quite likely that some of the physical symptoms associated with the illness can be equally affected by your mental attitude to them, and there's accumulating evidence that the body's immune system can be either improved or weakened by the effects of 'the psyche'. This is not to say that M.E. is a purely psychosomatic disease, one where the physical symptoms are *largely* under the control of the mind. But there is, for some sufferers, a psychosomatic element to their M.E., just as in other physical illnesses like asthma, where both physical factors (infections and allergies) can combine with emotional ones to exacerbate or cause relapse.

The relationship between the brain and the immune system is highly complex, and only just beginning to be understood by scientists interested in the subject – the study of what's now referred to as psychoneuroimmunology. It's not only the mind that can have an effect on body matter. The reverse process can also occur – what's known as somatopsychic illness, where the physical symptoms start to affect the emotional state, causing anxiety and depression as additional problems. These inter-relationships between mind and body are highly complicated, but in illnesses like M.E. they both probably occur in varying degrees of severity.

How can this knowledge be usefully applied to helping someone who's actually ill with M.E.? The obvious first step must be to try and take a 'positive approach'. I know it's not easy being optimistic when everything seems to be going wrong, but it's essential not to let your mind slip into the 'I'm never going to get better' approach, even when things are at their lowest ebb. Patients with HIV infection (AIDS) are now being taught to 'think positive' ('body positive'), even to the extent of imagining that the cells of their immune systems are actually being released 'into battle' against the persisting HIV infection, and killing off the virus (a technique called 'imaging'). There's no scientific proof that this approach actually reverses any of the immunedeficiency changes seen in AIDS, but it does stimulate a very positive approach of mind. I'm not suggesting that everyone with M.E. should sit down and meditate about their immune system killing off their persisting enteroviral infection, but I am advocating that *all* M.E. patients take a very positive approach to getting better. You *can* and *will* get better from M.E., even if it takes a long time.

M.E. is a very individual illness, in its presentation, symptoms, the secondary problems it causes, and the way it progresses. If you sit down with a group of fellow sufferers each one will probably have a symptom or a problem that no one else has. This is why it's essential to take an individual approach to the management in each case.

In the early stages (and in the case of M.E. this means anything up to the first two years or so after the illness started) when M.E. may not have even been diagnosed by the doctor, it's possible to remain optimistic, hoping that the mysterious symptoms can and will go away by themselves, given time. However, if time goes on and the symptoms don't improve, anxieties will naturally increase, especially if doctors are still searching for a diagnosis. Then, the day finally arrives when the patient gets a positive diagnosis of M.E. and this often creates a sense of tremendous relief.

At last, someone has produced an explanation for all these bizarre symptoms, and you have a 'genuine illness': something to be believed by your general practitioner (hopefully), your family and your friends. You've now got some idea of what's going wrong with your body, why you feel so ill all the time, and the sort of actions you should be taking to try and recover. Most importantly, you're no longer quite so alone. There are an awful lot of others who are suffering in a similar manner, who also find a trip to the supermarket a major effort, and have equal difficulties with friends and family when they're 'non-visibly' disabled.

However, this feeling of relief may only be temporary. After the diagnosis has been made, and the resulting consequences have started to sink in, a further change in attitude may then start to occur. Unfortunately, at this point, it's quite easy to become depressed and pessimistic about what may lie ahead. You start to realise that you're going to have to come to terms with the possibility of M.E. being a chronic illness, with the eventual outcome unpredictable, even to those who are looking after you. Both you and your family are now going to have to consider making very significant changes in lifestyle.

All kinds of questions will now arise: what to do about work, whether to put off starting or adding to the family, whether or not to move home. Making the correct decisions isn't going to be easy. At this point it's often very helpful to arrange to spend some time talking on a one-to-one basis with another M.E. sufferer, who can give sensible practical advice about 'living with M.E.', which your doctor can't do. Then, hopefully, you can keep in touch, even if it's only by phone or letter – with someone who really understands how you feel, and can offer sound advice when nobody else seems to know what to do.

If you're in an occupation such as teaching or nursing, talking to a fellow sufferer in the same job about how to cope with difficulties at work or with sick leave, can also be very helpful, just as mothers with young children can pick up equally useful advice from others in the same position. If you're having difficulty finding someone in the same occupation the M.E. Association may be able to help (see pages 196–8).

If you're having trouble with social security benefits, then talking to someone else who's experienced the same difficulties and won in the end can be very supporting. Try not to get fed up and give up. It doesn't help you, and it won't help other M.E. sufferers in the same situation in the future.

You may also be wondering about whether to start or extend a family. M.E. comes along at an age when this sort of decision is often about to be made. If a woman has M.E., this can be a very difficult decision to make – just how long should one keep putting off getting pregnant, whilst hoping that significant recovery is going to occur? Once again, talking things through with someone else who's got M.E. and become pregnant is the most useful advice that can be offered. (Pregnancy and M.E. is also covered on pages 127–31.)

At times when things aren't going too well, or you're going through a relapse or exacerbation of symptoms, try to think of this as being a set-back on the road to recovery – something that's only going to be temporary, which you *will* get over, and not an irreversible change for the worse.

STRESS, ANXIETY AND DEPRESSION

There's no doubt that although M.E. is capable of producing a wide range of psychiatric and emotional problems, the illness itself is definitely *not* a psychiatric disorder. For a few patients, psychiatric and emotional problems can become an increasingly distressing part of their illness, and when the doctors and specialists have missed the diagnosis of M.E. these aspects may even start to dominate their lives.

Some patients, with classic M.E. symptoms, are still being referred in desperation to psychiatrists by their general practitioners who feel there can be no other explanation. Fortunately, many of these patients do return from the visit with a clean bill of mental health, along with the comment that 'X isn't psychiatrically ill. There's something going wrong, but I don't know what it is.'

Understandably, depression is quite common in M.E. patients. Non-sufferers who are depressed are very commonly 'tired' as well, but this isn't the type of overwhelming exercise-related muscular fatigue and weakness experienced in M.E. The brain malfunction problems of M.E., such as loss of concentration and short-term memory, can also form part of depression, but mixing up words, carrying out inappropriate actions, lack of co-ordination and clumsiness related to physical or mental exertion are not characteristic of a depressive illness.

The final part of the M.E. symptom triad – the problems with autonomic nerve malfunction – are, as described earlier, thought to be due to overactivity of the sympathetic nerves. Unfortunately, these are also the nerves that can overact as part of acute anxiety, so some of the symptoms can be very similar in both conditions. Complaints such as palpitations, sweating, feeling tense or faint are common to both, and if prominent in M.E., the diagnosis of pure anxiety may be made. Again, there shouldn't be any confusion when the classic symptoms of muscle fatigue are added in, and the unusual problems of temperature control experienced in M.E. are not seen with anxiety.

One particular feature which does seem to be a true part of the M.E. disease process is what doctors refer to as emotional lability. Here, the patient's emotional state and mood may fluctuate widely, often for no apparent reason, but sometimes related to the frustrations imposed by the condition. Patients may suddenly burst into tears, feel extremely low and depressed or become uncharacteristically irritable with their family and friends. Not all M.E. patients experience these sorts of mood swing, but they can even occur in patients who would have regarded themselves as being very stable individuals, not subject to showing emotions, before the onset of their M.E.

It's important to remember that it's a perfectly normal human reaction to periodically feel very fed up with M.E., especially when you seem to be going through a bad patch, either due to the symptoms or associated problems at work or with your family. Who wouldn't, with such a frustrating condition which was imposing so many restrictions on your life? The important thing is to be able to differentiate being fed up from being truly depressed, and not letting all your feelings of inner anger radiate out and make everyone around you feel fed up as well.

Why do some M.E. patients go on to develop significant emotional and psychiatric problems, whereas others don't? The most important underlying reason is probably connected with previous personality, before M.E. ever arrived. By this we mean to what extent you used to be a 'coper' – how you used to react to life's major upsets and crises. Those who were used to 'sailing through' before, not letting things get them down too much, and having a generally optimistic view of life and the future are probably going to fare much better from the emotional point of view than the opposite type of personality. For people who do not cope as well, the problems associated with having M.E. may well tip the balance and trigger any underlying susceptibility to developing anxiety or a depressive illness – especially if this has already occurred in the past.

There is some evidence that women sufferers are more likely to succumb to these aspects of M.E., especially when they're part of a conventional family grouping. They may be quite unable to take time off to rest when they are still trying to cope with bringing up the children, doing the housework, and providing meals at the end of the day. Such women just don't get any chance to start the recovery process.

In contrast, the conventional husband who develops M.E. is still likely to be at work, and if he then goes on sick leave problems with the children and the home can be delegated while he initiates the major changes in lifestyle so necessary for recovery.

So, the M.E. patient's underlying personality may be the central factor in deciding how he or she manages to cope with

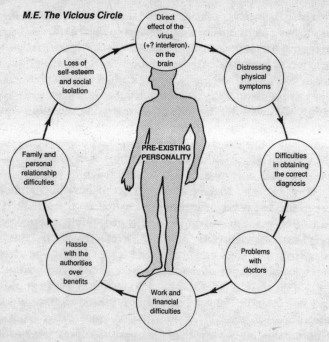

M.E. The Vicious Circle

Direct effect of the virus (+? interferon) on the brain

Distressing physical symptoms

Loss of self-esteem and social isolation

PRE-EXISTING PERSONALITY

Difficulties in obtaining the correct diagnosis

Family and personal relationship difficulties

Hassle with the authorities over benefits

Problems with doctors

Work and financial difficulties

this illness. Unfortunately, many other aspects of the condition may then start to interact and form a vicious circle which exacerbates the basic emotional problems.

Initiating this circle of events is the fact that the actual disease process in M.E. – the persisting viral infection – may be having a direct effect on parts of the brain which control emotion and mood, particularly the frontal lobes (see pages 38–42). It's already well known that an important cause of a true depressive illness is the aftermath of a viral infection. One possible explanation is that levels of neurotransmitters in key areas of the brain may be at fault, and secondly, the persisting virus may be causing the continued production of excess interferon, a substance which seems capable of having direct effects on various aspects of mental functioning.

Proceeding round the circle, the frustrating and disabling physical symptoms, and the constant feeling of being unwell are depressing in themselves. This can only then be increased in those who are still trying to get a diagnosis. The circle is completed, as time goes on, by the social, family and financial problems which so commonly become part of M.E., and these in turn aren't helped by battles with the authorities to obtain various sickness and disability benefits. All these social factors interact and may place a great strain, not only on the patient, but also his or her family. A resultant loss of self-esteem, even feelings of worthlessness, when all aspects of one's life seem to be falling apart, can place a tremendous pressure on the most stoic of individuals, and they may eventually find they just can't cope any longer.

So, it's not surprising that some M.E. patients pass from a state of just being 'fed up' from time to time, into true clinical depression, withdrawal from family and friends, and even have suicidal feelings. In severe cases such as this, the doctor may advise treatment with drugs.

TREATMENT OF DEPRESSION

In such cases as this, the doctor may advise treatment with drugs. These act by increasing those chemicals in the brain (neurotransmitters) which are thought to be depleted in depression. The most frequently prescribed are called tricyclic antidepressants, for which there are a large number of different trade names. These drugs can either be sedating (for a patient who has added anxiety or difficulty sleeping) or alerting (for patients who have also become very withdrawn and apathetic).

A common problem with all these drugs is their unpleasant side-effects, some of which can be very similar to pre-existing M.E. symptoms. They include gastric upsets, blurred vision, palpitations and weakness. They can be reduced by taking the tablets at night, and they do tend to diminish as time goes on.

Some newer drugs, called tetracyclics, may be a better alternative for M.E. patients. They seem to have fewer side-effects, although some doctors feel they are not quite as effective as the tricyclics.

With any antidepressant drug it's important to remember that they do have to be taken for a few weeks before providing any beneficial effects, and a proper course of treatment may last for several months.

When these antidepressant drugs do start to work the patient should start to sleep better, stop losing weight, and as mental activity once again quickens up the depressed mood starts to lift.

For a small group of M.E. patients their depression becomes quite incapacitating, a feeling of worthlessness gradually develops, even to the point of considering suicide as the only way out. At this stage professional psychiatric help is essential, possibly with a short period of hospital admission during this 'crisis period'. If you are feeling this low and there seems to be nobody you can talk to, do consider phoning the Samaritans (in the phone book), who may be able to offer some immediate help and advice.

ANXIETY

Anxiety is a common and quite normal response to any stressful situation. Many public performers have palpitations as they go on stage and anyone's pulse rate will rapidly rise if, for example, they have a near miss in traffic. It's only when these sort of symptoms become commonplace and out of all proportion to whatever the individual feels worried about that a state of anxiety exists.

As already mentioned, differentiating some of the symptoms of anxiety from M.E. may not be easy, even for an experienced doctor, and in those patients who are naturally prone to anxiety there may be a combination of both.

Common Symptoms of Anxiety

Psychological:
    Irritability and restlessness; difficulty getting to sleep
    Poor concentration
    Increased sensitivity to noise
Physical:
    Overactive autonomic nerves
        palpitations, sweating, diarrhoea, frequently passing urine, impotence
    From overbreathing (hyperventilation)
        dizziness, paraesthesiae ('pins and needles'), fainting
    From muscle spasm
        headaches, aches/tension in the neck or back

Some doctors are still far too keen on immediately treating any patient who has anxiety with a benzodiazepine tranquilliser such as diazepam (Valium). Such drugs act by dampening down nervous activity in the brain and in my experience at least half of all long-term M.E. sufferers have been given these sort of drugs to try at some stage in their illness.

On the whole these drugs should be avoided in M.E.; they have *no* effect whatsoever on the underlying disease process, and as they 'numb the mind' still further and exacerbate fatigue they may well make things worse. The only time to consider using them is for a very short period (i.e. days, not weeks or months) to deal with an acutely stressful event. Using them to blot out stress or anxiety is *not* a solution in M.E., and can lead to the problem of long-term dependence.

There are still far too many M.E. patients taking these drugs on a long-term basis, and in most cases this isn't helping them to recover from M.E. Once you've taken them for more than a few weeks, it is hard to stop, as many patients experience a withdrawal syndrome, very similar to the withdrawal problems seen with other drugs like alcohol, or even heroin. Many of the original symptoms of anxiety return as soon as there's no trace of the tranquilliser left in the body. As well, some of the withdrawal feelings can be very disturbing and frightening, such as increased sensitivity to noise, feelings of depersonalisation or being 'unreal', and occasionally hallucinations and delusions. Unfortunately these feelings can persist for weeks or months and be quite unbearable, so it is tempting for both doctor and patient to just restart the drug again.

Any M.E. patient who is taking long-term tranquillisers should seriously consider taking steps to 'come off', but as this withdrawal process isn't easy it must be done under medical supervision, and if your general practitioner isn't keen to help it may be necessary to ask for the advice of a psychiatrist. Self-help groups such as TRANX (see page 212 for address) can also provide counselling, and put you in touch with someone locally who has been through the withdrawal process. The dose must be reduced very slowly – over a period of four to twelve weeks, sometimes longer – to lessen any rebound anxiety taking place. Using one of the beta-blocking drugs during this withdrawal period can also help to reduce some of these unpleasant rebound anxiety symptoms. If drug treatment is really thought to be necessary for a patient with anxiety – especially if there are a lot of symptoms connected with autonomic overactivity – one of the beta-blocking drugs may be a possible alternative approach to a benzodiazepine (such as Valium), but they must be prescribed at the lowest dose possible.

However, a better approach to managing stress and anxiety is by self-help relaxation techniques, by which patients are able, themselves, to relax both body and mind – what one M.E. patient I know refers to as a 'dose of instant Valium'! You can discover how to do this from reading, learning from a cassette tape, or going to a relaxation class, but it does have to be carried out on a regular basis to be effective. Relaxation techniques can also be of help when getting to sleep is a problem.

Other techniques involving relaxation (e.g. meditation) are discussed on pages 171–2.

A GENERAL RELAXATION TECHNIQUE

- Set aside a quiet period each day, preferably for about twenty minutes or so twice a day, when you know you're not going to be disturbed.
- Sit comfortably in your favourite chair, or lie down quietly on the bed. Take the phone off the hook as well, to prevent any interruptions.
- Close your eyes, relax, and take in slow deep breaths at a regular pace. Don't overbreathe though!
- Allow your mind to wander on to some pleasant thought, sound or experience – whatever you feel appropriate. Listening to some tranquil music at the same time can be very soothing.
- **For muscular tension** This can be particularly useful for dealing with areas of muscular tension in the neck, and shoulders, etc., when associated with stress. However, it's not advisable to follow this part of the method for muscles which are painful and weak purely as a result of M.E.

    Learning to tense an area of muscle to the point of maximum tension and then having to relax it can be very beneficial. First, make a firm clenched fist with your hands, and notice the feeling of tension in the area. Then, let the fist suddenly relax and see how a warm heavy feeling then follows – indicating that it's now become fully relaxed. This process can be repeated in other 'trouble spots' around the body where muscle spasm/tension seems to be a problem, using the same principle of artificially producing tension followed by sudden relaxation.

By the end of the session you should now be feeling totally relaxed, and your breathing should be slow and regular. Have a few minutes doing nothing and then get up again. If you're using these techniques to help you get off to sleep at night they can be carried out shortly before retiring.

Relaxation tape cassettes can be obtained from the British Holistic Medical Association or Relaxation for Living, who also organise relaxation classes throughout the country (see pages 200 and 211).

Patients with anxiety problems may also find other alternative approaches such as yoga or meditation equally helpful.

PANIC ATTACKS

For those M.E. sufferers who already experience anxiety, panic attacks can be a further incapacitating pr 'lem. These attacks are brought on by fear, which is out of all proportion to the stressful situation.

Fears of going into public places or crowds of people in the course of using public transport or shopping in a busy supermarket (agoraphobia) are common causes. In some severe cases an attack can be caused simply by the fear of going out of the house.

To appreciate what such an attack feels like imagine how it feels when you've just stepped off the kerb and nearly been knocked down by a bus – a panic attack produces exactly the same sort of symptoms, but not for just a few seconds. The incapacity can last for up to half an hour. During such an attack a victim will feel unreal and start to tremble and shake inside. This is invariably accompanied by palpitations, chest pains and shortness of breath – even a feeling of choking. This rapid overbreathing (hyperventilation) washes out the carbon dioxide from the blood and causes the sensation of pins and needles (paraesthesiae) in the skin. Other common accompanying symptoms may include dizziness, sweating or flushing. Once the attack is over the patient feels thoroughly exhausted and apprehensive. These symptoms are produced by the autonomic nervous system suddenly becoming overactive when a patient is confronted by what they fear most.

The solution of panic attacks requires expert professional help. The benzodiazepine tranquillisers are best avoided, as in anxiety, but antidepressant medication can be quite helpful. Drug treatment, however, won't succeed by itself, and patients have to learn to control their bodies, especially the over-breathing during an attack. The relaxation techniques already described to help anxiety may also be useful here, and a further approach known as behaviour therapy can also be tried.

Behaviour therapy involves the patient being gradually exposed to the sort of situations they fear. In the case of crowds and open spaces this may firstly involve just looking at pictures and thinking about the situations for short periods. This is then followed by short trips outside the house in the company of a friend or counsellor, until eventually the patient feels confident enough to confront what they fear most. This is a slow, time-consuming approach, which requires practical assistance from an experienced therapist, but when carried out can be very effective in reducing phobic anxiety. Further self-help can be obtained from the Phobic Society (see page 210).

PART 2
PRACTICAL STEPS TOWARDS COPING WITH M.E.

1. M.E. And Your Doctor

My personal experiences over the past few years, both as a doctor and as an M.E. sufferer, have made me appreciate the fact that in many chronic diseases doctors only play a relatively small role in any recovery process. What is far more important in conditions like M.E. is how patients learn to help themselves, and the actions which other individuals and agencies can carry out, both to help and hinder recovery. When doctors discuss the management of such conditions they tend to concentrate on the medical side of the treatment, often failing to take into account the humanising factors which are so important when trying to cope with something like M.E. So, unless the patient, the illness, the family, and the environment are all taken into consideration progress won't be made. Fortunately, many doctors are now becoming increasingly convinced that this holistic approach to illness, where the humanising aspects are regarded as being equally important as the purely medical treatment, is a far better way of managing patients with conditions like M.E.

The current trend towards high-tech medicine has also falsely raised the expectations of many patients, as to what doctors can actually do in 'curing' disease. The attitude the patient takes towards his or her illness is going to be far more important. A positive approach to recovery, making appropriate changes in lifestyle, sympathetic support from doctors, family and friends are all essential components.

Equally, external factors will all have an important role to play in the recovery process, and if M.E. patients are battling to obtain social service benefits, or having to give up their jobs because they can no longer cope, this will obviously have a very adverse effect on the outcome.

In any disease where doctors and orthodox medicine are at present so limited in the help they can offer, it's hardly surprising that many patients are keen to try one of the numerous alternative approaches, and these are dealt with in detail on pages 154–74.

GETTING M.E. DIAGNOSED BY YOUR DOCTOR

Why do some doctors find it so difficult to cope with their M.E. patients, their diagnosis and management? It's very instructive to place yourself in their position. In order to understand how your doctor sees you – the patient with M.E. – it's necessary to go right back to the onset of your M.E.

Your first consultation was probably along the lines: 'I had this dose of flu a few weeks ago, but I'm definitely *not* getting over it. I'm tired all the time, and I've got tired, aching muscles which soon get weak after exercise, and then my brain won't work either.'

At this point the GP's role is essentially trying to work out some sort of 'label' for your condition. If he can do that, he can then suggest some form of management, which may be via the prescription pad. Your doctor would very much like to 'cure' the condition which has just been diagnosed, but if that's not possible at least try to alleviate some of the symptoms. If he can't decide what's wrong, and you don't seem to have any complaints which suggest something seriously wrong, he may well conclude it's a 'self-limiting condition', i.e. it will go away in its own time. And, like so many patients he sees – where it's not possible to make a firm diagnosis – he'll be hoping that both you and your strange symptoms will now go away without any further investigations or treatment!

Now, if doctors can't actually recognise a particular pattern of symptoms and associate them with a specific disease, they're not going to diagnose that condition, and that's why so many sufferers come unstuck at the first hurdle – getting a diagnosis. Patients who present with characteristic M.E. symptoms will find that their GP is all too familiar with them as individual symptoms, but put them all together and he's probably quite baffled, unless he's already become aware of M.E.

At this point the patient is often informed that 'You've got a bit of "post-viral debility", or "post-flu flop"; take it easy for a while and you'll soon feel better.' In fact, if you have got M.E., it's really crucial in this very early stage that you should now be in bed resting, for it seems that this may well have a very positive effect on your chances of recovery. Far too many M.E. patients return to work or household and family duties, struggle on, and make their condition gradually worse until they can't cope any longer.

On the second or third visits you're 'still not well', can't cope with your normal daily routine or work, sleeping whenever you can, and you've got the characteristic overwhelming muscle fatigue and brain malfunction.

With all these persisting symptoms how does the doctor go about trying to make a diagnosis? They have to rely on key pieces of information – medical clues.

The first key piece of information comes from what you tell the doctor – what's known as your clinical history – and in general practice this is where the most important clues come from. If the diagnosis of M.E. isn't fairly obvious to the doctor after a patient has given a good description of M.E., then information from the rest of the consultation isn't likely to provide the answer.

The second part of the assessment, the physical examination, may well reinforce the doctor's belief that you're not physically unwell, because he or she may find the patient's muscle power relatively normal. Only the astute physician who goes to the bother of exercising an M.E. sufferer to the point of fatigue will find that muscle weakness does indeed occur.

Doctors who are prepared to thoroughly examine their patients, may well find, as Dr Melvin Ramsay has repeatedly observed, that very careful fingertip palpation of particular muscles (especially the trapezius in the neck and the gastrocnemius in the leg) can demonstrate tiny foci of exquisite tenderness. Unfortunately, this art of clinical examination is all too often being replaced by spending time looking at bits of paper from the laboratory.

M.E. patients also complain of unsteadiness. Doctors use a test to assess this symptom (Romberg's test), where they ask you to try and stand still with the eyes closed. The results of this may be quite normal. Unsteadiness is a very common symptom which GPs deal with frequently, but if they can't find an obvious cause they may think anxiety, only, is the cause.

BLOOD TESTS

Your doctor may next decide to see if any abnormalities show up in blood tests. With M.E. sufferers these routine blood tests often come back from the lab relatively normal, so their value is partly in excluding other possible causes for the symptoms.

Typical blood tests which your GP may carry out include:

The ESR (erythrocyte sedimentation rate) Healthy individuals have red blood cells which do not tend to stick together. However, in a wide range of illnesses – particularly infections and inflammatory conditions – this stickiness increases so that the cells clump together (agglutinate) and hence sediment more easily.

The ESR test measures the speed at which such sedimentation occurs, and if raised indicates that 'something is wrong somewhere'. In M.E. the ESR is almost always within the normal range (which may be significant in view of the Australian findings on blood cell shape described on page 12) and this may suggest to the doctor that the patient has no serious health problem.

Haemoglobin (Hb) contains the iron in the blood, and if decreased, shows if any anaemia is present. M.E. patients shouldn't be anaemic – if you are there must be some other cause apart from M.E., and this requires further investigation by your doctor.

White Blood Count (WBC) measures the number of cells in the blood which are primarily produced to fight infections. There are several different types including neutrophils, lymphocytes and eosinophils. In the early stage of an infection the lymphocytes are often raised in number – a lymphocytosis. As the condition becomes chronic there may be no significant abnormalities, even though the virus is persisting, although a few patients do then seem to show a decrease in their white cell counts. Sometimes M.E. patients have a few abnormally shaped lymphocytes under the microscope, suggesting the presence of persisting infection. T lymphocytes can't be seen on this sort of routine blood examination requested by a GP. They need to be done at specialist centres.

Immunoglobulins are the antibodies in the blood, and minor changes in the levels of IgA and IgM are sometimes seen.

Enzymes are proteins which are released from inside a cell when inflammation or damage occurs. The different body tissues all produce their own characteristic enzymes which can easily be measured once they spill into the blood, so the actual site(s) of damage can often be identified. Coxsackie infections can sometimes inflame the liver (hepatitis) during the early stages of M.E., so specific liver enzymes might be found using a blood test.

Muscle enzymes are also released into the blood in a variety of muscle diseases. Creatine kinase is the one most frequently measured, but only about 5 or 10 per cent of M.E. patients have raised levels, usually early on in the illness. Unfortunately, having a normal muscle enzyme profile may yet again lead the doctor to the assumption that there is nothing wrong in the muscle.

Thyroid function tests Some doctors will also want to check the function of the thyroid gland. There are two reasons for this.

Firstly, in an older patient, partial failure of the gland may already be occurring and this can produce a range of symptoms which have many similarities to those of M.E., e.g. fatigue, muscle aches, poor brain function, etc. (If there is any co-existent thyroid malfunction it is likely to make any M.E. symptoms worse.) Secondly, although rare, the Coxsackie viruses are capable of causing an inflammation of the thyroid gland which in the early stages causes overactivity (hyperthyroidism) and may then be followed by underactivity (hypothyroidism or myxoedema) – although the latter usually resolves in time.

Even after doing all these investigations the doctor may still be left with a diagnostic problem: a patient whose symptoms he doesn't recognise; nothing to find wrong on examination; and a whole series of normal laboratory results. If the doctor is alert to the possibility of M.E. he may then decide to look for evidence of persisting viral infection.

TESTING FOR THE PRESENCE OF PERSISTING VIRAL INFECTION

There is still no definitive test for M.E. – what we do have are further blood tests which either show the presence of antibodies to enteroviruses such as Coxsackie B, or the new 'VP1 test', which if positive, demonstrates the presence of a persisting enterovirus.

The antibody tests merely state that the body has reacted in the past (neutralising antibodies) or is probably still reacting (IgM antibodies) to the Coxsackie virus. Although providing useful information, these tests are of limited value, and even when positive don't 'prove' someone has M.E., and at the same time if negative won't disprove the diagnosis.

The VP1 Test VP1 stands for Viral Protein One. It is one of four different proteins which form the outer capsule of any enterovirus. One specific portion of VP1 is present in *all* of the seventy-two different enteroviruses.

The researchers at St Mary's Hospital, London, have developed an antibody which can identify this common portion of VP1 and have used it to develop this blood test. A positive test indicates the presence of enterovirus in the blood, but not which one. It is *not* a 'test for M.E.' or an indicator of disease activity. It can also be positive in someone who has picked up an enteroviral infection and just has a cold, so it has to be interpreted with caution. As far as M.E. is concerned a positive test will support the diagnosis, and in patients tested so far, about 55 per cent are positive. A negative result does not exclude the diagnosis of M.E., but means another type of virus (possibly Epstein–Barr) is responsible. If you are already diagnosed there is no necessity to have this test done, but if the diagnosis is in doubt it may be helpful.

The VP1 test is not available, as yet, from local hospital laboratories. If your GP thinks the test is relevant you should then get in touch with the M.E. Association (see pages 196–8) who will send you full details as well as a blood testing pack (there is a small fee for this). Your GP can then take the sample, which is analysed at St Mary's, and the result comes back to your GP.

OTHER TESTS USED IN M.E.

The very important findings being obtained from muscle biopsies, single fibre EMGs and nuclear magnetic resonance studies, were discussed previously.

Again, these investigations are not diagnostic tests for M.E. They are presently research based and only used in a few teaching hospital centres in the U.K., and require the expertise of specialists to carry them out. For these reasons they are not generally available, and patients with M.E. are unlikely to be referred for any of them, unless they are seeing a specialist involved in a particular research project.

GETTING THE DIAGNOSIS WRONG

Unfortunately, due to doctors' unfamiliarity with M.E., and because there are no precise methods for diagnosing it, many

M.E. sufferers have had to wait years for a correct diagnosis. Invariably the stories are the same: loads of tests often repeated, visits to baffled physicians, neurologists and psychiatrists, nobody can decide 'what's wrong', and eventually the doctor gives up. It's not therefore surprising that some patients don't want to see another doctor ever again, and their faith in the medical profession has been severely undermined.

If a doctor doesn't recognise the patient's muscular symptoms as being due to M.E. his first thoughts may be to consider another type of neurological disease. I know many patients who have initially been diagnosed as having multiple sclerosis or had extensive investigations for myasthenia gravis. When these investigations fail to support the diagnosis, and the symptoms don't follow the expected pattern, some neurologists give up and pass the patient back to the GP with no firm diagnosis. The patient still has M.E. symptoms, the neurologist decides there's nothing more he can do, so the next step is for the GP to request a psychiatrist's opinion. Although tiredness and fatigue are a common part of a depressive illness the muscular fatigue and 'recovery period' are unique features of M.E. Most alert psychiatrists seem to be able to recognise the fact that M.E. sufferers are not 'psychiatrically ill', but a few patients are not so lucky, get labelled as being depressed, and then it's extremely difficult to change such an opinion.

Again, some of the symptoms of M.E. can be very similar to those of acute anxiety, and there are a few such patients who have been wrongly diagnosed as having M.E., when they have a form of anxiety known as chronic hyperventilation – where overbreathing causes fatigue and various other symptoms. The reverse is probably also true.

Lastly it's important, where anyone suspected of having M.E. has agricultural connections, to exclude chronic infections such as brucellosis and toxoplasmosis, some of whose symptoms can be very close to M.E. For anyone working on a dairy farm or in contact with contaminated water (such as canoeists and anglers with open cuts) the organism Leptospira hardjo can cause a flu-like illness followed by persisting malaise and severe headaches. It's very important that this is recognised and treated right away with an antibiotic.

CONDITIONS WHICH CAN BE MISTAKEN FOR M.E.	
Neurological Disease	Myasthenia Gravis
	Multiple Sclerosis
Psychiatric Illness	Depression
	Hyperventilation Syndrome
Chronic Infections	Brucellosis and Lyme Disease
(may be treatable)	Toxoplasmosis
	Leptospirosis Hardjo
Rheumatic Disorders	Fibromyalgia
Glandular Disorders	Hypothyroidism (Myxoedema)
	Addison's Disease (failure of the adrenal gland)

HOW TO DEAL WITH YOUR DOCTOR ONCE M.E. IS DIAGNOSED

M.E. sufferers don't make easy patients – you've got what is probably a long-term illness that can't be 'cured'; you have a wide variety of symptoms which modern medicine is very limited in its ability to help, and you may also have a whole range of social, emotional and employment problems which require help. So, from your GP's point of view M.E. patients are not the easiest of people to manage successfully.

Despite all these hurdles, an increasing number of doctors are becoming interested in M.E. and consequently diagnosing the illness correctly in the vital early stages. Unfortunately, some doctors still remain ignorant of the recent research advances. So, if you are convinced that M.E. is the cause of your symptoms don't be fobbed off with explanations that 'the disease does not exist', and try to obtain an opinion from a doctor who is aware of the condition.

Some physicians are becoming increasingly aware and in-volved in what is termed the holistic approach to medicine and patient care. This means they take into account not only your physical illness, but also your attitude to it, the interaction between you and your family and any environmental factors which may be having an effect.

It's this sort of approach, where everything is considered, and the patient's family fully involved, that is particularly appropriate to conditions like M.E.

REFERRAL TO CONSULTANTS

Is there any need for you to be referred to a consultant? Obviously, yes, if your general practitioner has any doubt about the diagnosis. But as many patients know from bitter experience, this can still be counter productive, and even harmful if you then end up seeing a specialist who isn't familiar with M.E. The diagnosis is missed and thoughts of a 'psychiatric problem' then become foremost in the GP's mind. Having had one specialist opinion who 'can't find anything wrong' your GP may then feel very reluctant to send you to other specialists for further second opinions, and so the psychiatrist becomes the only option. And so the merry-go-round of general physician–neurologist–psychiatrist goes on till someone finally makes the correct diagnosis.

As M.E. symptoms cross a whole range of medical boundaries (virology, infectious diseases, neurology, gut problems, immunology, etc.) specialists in a wide range of subjects have become involved. It should now be possible, in most parts of the country, to find a specialist interested in M.E., although this may mean travelling to the local teaching hospital.

Your own GP may know of a local specialist interested in M.E., but if he doesn't there'll be an element of pot luck involved, if you're just referred to a local general physician. One useful source of information in these circumstances are members of the local M.E. group, who are often very well informed about who's worth going to see – and not worth going to see.

Consultants don't generally like seeing patients privately unless they're first referred by their GP, so it's always best to ask your family doctor to write a referral note. Some GPs actually get very upset when their patients go off to see private consultants without their knowledge or 'permission' – and they do have a valid point. Even if a consultant is prepared to see you without a referral letter, it's still regarded as being unethical if they don't then keep your GP fully informed about their diagnostic opinion or treatment.

If you're really not happy about the way your GP is managing your illness, do think very carefully about going off for other opinions without discussing it, as it's quite likely to put an additional strain on your relationship.

In Britain, there's nothing to prevent your GP referring you on to an NHS specialist outside your usual health district, although many hospitals actively discourage such referrals. The other problem in doing so is that those specialists who are interested in M.E., particularly in London, have at times become so overwhelmed by such requests, that they've become practically unable to cope with any further outside requests.

M.E. really is a condition which is ideally managed by good and interested general practitioners – provided you can find them.

UNINTERESTED DOCTORS

What can you do if your general practitioner just isn't interested or sympathetic towards M.E., and can't accept that you really do feel as ghastly as you claim?

Your doctor may well be one of those who is just not interested in chronic illnesses, where there's very little he can do to alleviate the symptoms or change the course of the disease by writing out something on the prescription pad. He may be one of those doctors who doesn't really like talking to his patients for more than ten minutes, and feels that emotional problems aren't his concern – whereas for the patient they're an extremely important part of the illness.

If you have got a doctor in this category, and his attitude doesn't seem to change, even after you've gone to the bother of getting him all the latest medical references on the subject, there's probably no other option but to try and find someone else. If you belong to a group practice it should be quite easy to see another partner, and you may not have to actually change on to their individual list. Any good practice should have a flexible policy for patients who find they don't have any rapport with their doctor and want to see another member of the team.

Alternatively, you might try the practice 'trainee' if they have one – a good sign that the practice has come up to standard when it was selected for such a purpose. Trainee general practitioners are often bright young doctors, fresh from doing three or four years in hospital medicine, but are now intending to enter general practice. They work for an introductory year under the supervision of one of the senior partners in the practice. Trainees often have more time to devote to their individual patients, and are often encouraged to take on unusual or 'difficult' conditions – even writing them up as part of their examination – so if you find a trainee taking considerable time and interest in your case, stick with him or her. Unfortunately, they're only with the practice for one year, and only rarely progress on to a job in the same practice, so this isn't a long-term solution.

As a last resort you may have to consider finding another GP altogether. Try and find out from friends and neighbours (or other M.E. sufferers) about the local doctors, and possibly go round and ask if the one you choose is prepared to take you on to the list. Some doctors are even quite happy for prospective patients to come to the surgery for a quick chat before joining the practice.

In Britain, however, it's worth remembering that the GP is paid on a capitation fee system – about £8 every year for each patient on the list, no matter how many times he sees or visits you – so there's no great incentive to encourage people with chronic illnesses to join the list!

As many M.E. patients are already too well aware, some doctors tend to be very wary of patients who 'swap' doctors in the same area, and may view you as a potential problem. Also, practices have fairly well-defined geographical limits on who they're prepared to take on, so outside large towns such action may be practically very difficult or even impossible.

If you do decide to change doctor try not to leave it to your Family Practitioner Committee to allocate you a new practice. This really is the last resort, and a very bad start to any new doctor–patient relationship. No doctor likes having patients allocated to them by an anonymous administrator, whether they like it or not. Your local Community Health Council or FPC can help you further with the technical details of how to change, and the local post office and library should have a full list of all local general practitioners.

The final option is to opt out of the NHS altogether and go privately, but do take advice and think very carefully about who you go and see, or you could end up spending a lot of money on unnecessary drugs and investigations and just getting the wrong advice. In many large towns there are now a few purely private general practitioners, but you're not supposed to remain on an NHS practitioner's list at the same time. A private GP, although he may obviously be able to spend more time with you, may not know any more about M.E. than your NHS one.

There aren't any easy answers about how to establish a good doctor–patient relationship; a lot depends on pure luck and where you happen to live. At the end of the day it's like any relationship – some doctors just don't hit it off with some of their patients and vice versa. You've really got to treat it like a marriage – if both partners don't contribute it won't work.

2. M.E. And Your Job

One of the most urgent problems facing many M.E. sufferers can be trying to adjust financially to the limitations imposed by the illness.

Where the sufferer has been the main breadwinner, and is also quite young, with rapidly rising financial and promotional expectations from work, the loss of income can be abrupt and severe. A large mortgage might have been taken out on a new house, or other costly financial planning entered into, and now these commitments may be impossible to keep going. Even the most fortunate individuals (in Britain) are unlikely to receive more than six months' full sick pay and an equal period of half pay. After that, the total family income may rapidly diminish to a combination of state sickness benefits, and whatever other members of the family are bringing in. And, where a wife is at home looking after small children, this may mean no other source of earned income.

A financial crisis may then ensue, forcing sudden decisions to cut back on spending. It's far preferable to try and avoid this by talking to one's bank manager or building society before such a crisis occurs, to put them in the picture, and hopefully make some arrangements to ease the burden in the short term.

This chapter is designed to give practical help and advice on the sorts of problem which occur, and the options to consider in trying to solve them. It applies not only to difficulties with employment but also to the large number, and complex rules governing eligibility for DHSS benefits.

PROBLEMS AT WORK

In the early stages of the illness, often before a firm diagnosis has been made, employers tend to be fairly sympathetic to a sufferer's condition, but this approach tends to rapidly evaporate as the months pass by, and your absence becomes a steadily increasing inconvenience. There comes a time when the employer begins to wonder if you're ever going to return to work. Just how long can this persisting virus go on? Unfortunately, neither you nor your doctor can provide them with the answers they require, and their impatience gets worse.

You may attempt to go back to work, even though you know you're almost certainly not well enough to do so. This attempt fails, and you end up feeling even more demoralised. The company then decides it's looking extremely unlikely that you're going to return in the near future, and the next thing you hear is that somebody else has been promoted into your position: there's no job to go back to even if you are well!

It's a popular misconception that you can't lose your job due to ill health – unfortunately this isn't so. After a prolonged period away from work your employer may be able to argue that this is a valid reason for dismissal.

The first important step, if you feel you're about to enter this situation, is to get in touch with your trade union or professional body, and talk to one of their industrial relations advisors. It's essential to take expert advice here, as the law is complicated, and these people should be fully up-to-date with the legislation, and be able to refer you on for appropriate legal advice if necessary. If you don't belong to such organisations the local Citizens Advice Bureau (in Britain) should be able to give you some help.

Secondly, do keep in touch with work (probably the personnel officer) and let them know what's happening about your progress, or lack of it – they may even be able to help financially. Admittedly, some employers are excellent when it comes to problems related to ill health, but others just don't want to know, and hope you'll quietly go away.

It's also worthwhile making an appointment with the company doctor, if you have an occupational health service, to keep him informed. If he's interested and sympathetic towards M.E., he may be able to offer help in the future, and his opinion will be important if it comes to taking early retirement on the grounds of ill health.

If you are claiming sick pay under an occupational sick pay scheme, dismissal shouldn't be a way of stopping such benefits, but again, check the law with your trade union.

DISMISSAL ON GROUNDS OF ILL HEALTH – GOING TO LAW

If it comes to the point of actually being dismissed because you've got M.E., there may be an internal company appeal procedure to which you or your trade union could present your case. Your employer may argue that your contract of employment has been terminated, because in the legal jargon, it has been 'frustrated'. (This means that your employer now considers that you are unable to perform your contractual duties due to continuing ill health with M.E.)

If you are dismissed, and all appeals to the company have failed, you may still have a case which could be taken to an industrial tribunal – but you *must* do this within three months of dismissal. The industrial tribunal will have to decide if your employer was acting in a 'fair and reasonable manner' when they decided to terminate employment. You may think that it's very unfair to be dismissed through no actual fault of your own, and a tribunal may agree with you if you can successfully argue points such as:

- You were never in any way consulted about your illness and possible return to work by the employer.
- The employer never went to the bother of obtaining relevant medical reports on your state of health from either your doctor or their own occupational health physician.

The tribunal also has to take into account the fact that your ill health could be endangering other employees, and in the case of M.E., this could well be relevant where a manual worker is operating dangerous machinery, or somebody driving public transport.

Any M.E. sufferer who has registered as being disabled for the purposes of employment may find this gives some added protection against dismissal.

The law regarding employment and dismissal on grounds of ill health is very complex, so do get expert advice before you make any irretrievable decisions.

RETIREMENT ON GROUNDS OF ILL HEALTH

If you've been in a company pension or superannuation scheme and you decide to retire due to ill health, then some form of pension may now be payable. Unfortunately, a common problem is that the qualifying criterion for obtaining a pension, at a very early age, is 'permanent ill health' (i.e. you're not going to ever work again due to the illness). As the outcome in any individual case of M.E. is so unpredictable, especially in the first few years of the illness, no medical specialist is likely to firmly give the opinion that you're inevitably going to remain in a state of 'permanent ill health'. Consequently, the pension or award may then be frozen until it becomes clear that you are very likely to remain permanently disabled by M.E. – and this may be several years.

SOME OTHER OPTIONS WITH EMPLOYMENT

You may feel that if you've had to give up your job because of M.E. there's nothing else you can now do, but it is important to explore other possibilities.

It may be possible to arrange some part-time work in your previous type of occupation, or do some 'flexitime' to fit in with the times of day when you seem to function most productively. Another employer might be able to offer you a similar type of job, but at a less demanding pace, and probably at a less demanding salary. However, for many sufferers these sorts of option may not exist, or be practical, and then there's no choice but to rely on financial support from the various state sickness benefits.

Being at home all day, no longer making any decisions and missing out on the social life and friendships that are all part of 'being at work' is a very demoralising aspect of M.E., which often exacerbates the feelings of isolation and loss of self-esteem. It obviously depends on how unwell you are, what stage the illness is at, and how variable the symptoms are, but giving up work for good is one of the most difficult decisions to make in M.E., so *do* look at the other possibilities – state of health permitting.

SELF-EMPLOYMENT AND M.E.

One further practical possibility worth exploring is that of becoming self-employed and carrying on some form of work from home. This has some distinct attractions, as it can be very flexible, carried out at times when you're fit enough, and temporarily abandoned when you're unwell.

Obviously, this is an option for those M.E. sufferers who feel able, and want to continue with some form of work. I fully accept, that for many M.E. sufferers, what I'm suggesting just isn't going to be possible now, but it may be later on when you start to make progress. It's also important to appreciate that if you do continue to claim invalidity benefit, there may come a time when they will review your position. And, if they feel that despite being unable to perform your normal occupation, there is some 'suitable alternative work' you could do, this could be used as a reason to stop benefit.

Whatever you do decide to do about work, try not to make any hasty decisions – take time to consider all the options available, and take account of what other members of the family feel is right. And, don't ever resign from your job because of M.E. until you've first taken expert advice – you may end up disqualifying yourself from financial assistance.

There are no simple answers to the very common question: 'What do I do about my job?' It very much depends on the stage of the illness, what you do for a living, and the attitude of your employers and possibly the company doctor.

For those who have been diagnosed early on in the illness, a period of sick leave with complete rest, followed by gradual convalescence is the aim. Then perhaps a staged return to work, which will have to be flexible, and avoid excessive amounts of stress or overwork on any one day. Other patients who are diagnosed late, when the condition seems to have stabilised and possibly become chronic, may have much more difficult decisions to take. At this point little benefit is likely to be gained from prolonged bed rest. The choice may have to be between making a major readjustment in occupation or leaving the current type of occupation, if the physical and mental stresses are too much.

Unfortunately, the financial and psychological consequences of giving up work may also have their own negative effects on recovery in M.E. – unemployment can also damage your health. So, like all the other routes to recovery it's a question of trying to strike the right balance between the advantages and disadvantages, and at the same time keeping within your limitations.

It may not be easy to find such a person to talk to, but I always think it can be of immense help in these circumstances to listen to someone else in the same occupation as yourself who has M.E. and find out what they did. An M.E. self-help organisation may be able to put you in touch with someone.

Here is a quote from a recent article in the *Journal of the Society for Occupational Medicine*, by Dr Mike Peel, who is an Occupational Physician with British Airways. This is an account of the problems in returning to work which some of his patients with M.E. have faced, and is to be recommended to any other occupational health physicians.

The most important impression is that they are all very active, fit and dedicated workers: the last ones likely to exaggerate symptoms. Managers have expressed relief that a trusted colleague is genuinely ill and not hysterical. It is probable that the attitude of fighting on despite illness is a critical factor, in that they continued working long hours and taking regular exercise long after their bodies told them to stop.

J. Soc. Occup. Med. *(1988) 38, 44–5*

3. Running Your Home

The disabling physical symptoms of M.E. mean that many sufferers share the same sort of practical difficulties that other chronically disabled groups have in trying to lead a normal life. You're not alone in experiencing the sort of frustrations imposed by M.E. These may range from the pure physical inability to summon up sufficient strength to carry out a routine task like mowing the lawn, to difficulties with gripping or manipulating everyday objects used in the kitchen.

The combination of muscular fatigue and unsteadiness also produces great difficulty in coping with tasks that involve prolonged standing and concentrating. This not only prevents many sufferers following their normal occupations but it also makes many of the domestic tasks involved in running a home equally difficult.

To make life easier there are a number of practical aids available either free, on loan, or to buy, which will help to make many physical and manipulative tasks less fatiguing. There are also various professionals and agencies who can give invaluable help when it comes to learning to cope with disability (see Part 4, pages 175–95). It's perfectly natural to feel reluctant to label yourself as being 'disabled'. You don't have to use the term if you don't want to, but if you are having practical difficulties do make use of the resources which are available.

Before approaching anyone for help it's a good idea to make a comprehensive written list of the sort of practical problems with which you require help. This might be something as simple as obtaining a device which can open tight tops on the marmalade jar, to how you can obtain expert assistance and financial help in making major adaptations to the home for a very disabled M.E. sufferer. Don't be afraid to go round asking questions. The people involved are usually very approachable and only too willing to help.

If adapting your home involves making a claim for a benefit or grant don't be put off because you're not sure about your eligibility: as long as you provide the officials with honest information it can't do any harm. If you are then refused, but still think you have a good case, do make an appeal, as the success rate in challenging the bureaucracy over disabled benefits is quite high. In the meantime, there are many ways you can conserve your energy and make life easier.

IN THE HOME

Here are some practical suggestions, room by room.

Kitchens

- Keep commonly used foods and kitchen utensils together in an easily accessible place – preferably at chest height, to avoid repeated reaching up and bending down.
- Use level work surfaces for heavy objects: they can be pushed around instead of lifted.
- Raise the washing-up bowl in the sink so you're not stooping over, and let the washing-up dry by itself.
- If you can afford it, consider purchasing a dish-washing machine.
- Again, if you can afford it, consider other types of electrical apparatus which can make life easier: a microwave, a freezer to store some essential foods in, or an electric tin opener.
- There are numerous aids which make a whole range of domestic duties and cooking much easier, e.g. specially adapted cutlery and cooking utensils, plugs with small handles so they're easier to pull out of the socket, etc. Visit one of the disabled living centres (see page 204), and see what's on display that might help you.

Living rooms

- If you have difficulty getting out of a low chair or sofa due to weakness in the hip muscles, consider getting a comfortable high chair, or one with a raised seat.

- A sofa bed may be a very useful additional piece of furniture if you're frequently confined to bed for 'relapses', and don't like spending your time upstairs confined to the bedroom.

Stairs
- These can be a major problem for anyone who has been severely weakened by M.E., and may mean that a sufferer is confined to either the downstairs or upstairs for long periods. Chair lifts, although expensive, are a very useful device in such circumstances, but do take expert advice before spending large amounts of money: visit a disabled living centre for further practical help.
- If you do tend to live downstairs during a relapse, and sleep down there, it may be worth considering installing a downstairs toilet and shower.

Bathroom
- A hand rail, fixed to the wall by the bath, will help getting in and out.
- Buy a non-slip bath mat.
- Sitting in a shower can be less tiring than taking a bath. Use a special board across the bath top to sit on, but make sure it's stable and won't slip. (The Red Cross may loan you one.)
- Washing hair in the bath is a lot easier than bending over the sink.
- If your 'carer' is often having to lift you in and out of the bath, consider installing some form of hoist device.

Bedrooms
- Cut down on the bed-making by making use of fitted sheets and duvets.

OUT AND ABOUT – SHOPPING

- Local voluntary groups may be able to provide an able-bodied volunteer to help with a weekly shop, or a driver to take you there. Some schools also have volunteer sections.
- Find out about any local dial-a-ride services or other schemes to improve mobility.

- Consider alternatives to going out to the shops. Shopping from home can be done via mail order; some shops will still deliver groceries; and the milkman now carries an increasingly diverse range of produce.
- Ask a friend or neighbour to buy certain goods on a regular basis when they go to the supermarket.
- Find out about supermarkets and department stores which have special shopping hours reserved for the disabled; some also have priority parking facilities.
- Get the able-bodied members of the family (or friends) to buy certain items in bulk, as long as you have the storage space.
- Make sure that you've always got a stock of essential items of food, so that in a relapse when you can't get out for several days, there is something to eat.

4. Increasing Your Mobility

Problems with mobility are a major cause of social isolation for the disabled, as well as creating extra difficulties in obtaining employment, so do take advantage of any of the help that's available and appropriate to your own individual needs.

Pure financial help may be forthcoming from the social services in the form of a Mobility Allowance, but this isn't easy to qualify for. The Department of Employment can also help with fares to work (see Part 4).

WALKING AIDS

A walking stick will help to provide extra support, relieve muscle and joint pains, and increase mobility.

Make sure that the stick you buy is the correct length for your body – you shouldn't end up leaning towards the stick (too short) or away from it (too long). If the stick has a metal or wooden tip it can easily slip in wet weather. A soft rubber tip is the best way to increase the friction and grip, and just like the tyres on a car these rubber tips need to be changed when worn. Pyramid sticks have either three or four legs and may be helpful if you require a considerable amount of support. If you're out and about quite a bit, it might be worth buying a shooting stick which has a fold-up seat on the top.

For those who are severely disabled the Zimmer type of walking frame may be necessary – a physiotherapist will give you appropriate advice.

WHEELCHAIRS

Only a very few M.E. sufferers are ever likely to have to make use of a wheelchair, and this may be something which is used on a temporary rather than permanent basis to aid mobility during an arduous day's activities.

Wheelchairs can be obtained from a variety of sources.

1 From the DHSS Artificial Limb and Appliance Centre
Your doctor will have to complete a special assessment form in order to get one from this source. The best way of obtaining the model best suited to your individual needs is to make arrangements to visit a 'wheelchair clinic' at one of these centres, so your requirements can be assessed by an expert. You can also be visited at home for this assessment. Alternatively, a local physiotherapist or occupational therapist can help with the choice of the most appropriate model – and the DHSS has over 140 models available!

Wheelchairs from the DHSS are given on free loan. All the models which are available from the DHSS are described in the 'Handbook of Wheelchairs' (MM408) which is available from the DHSS store, Manchester Road, Heywood, Lancashire.

2 Purchased privately There are perfectly reputable private suppliers of wheelchairs, but do take advice first before spending large sums of money.

3 The British Red Cross is very willing to make short-term loans to those who just require extra help for a short period, e.g. when going on holiday. They also produce a useful leaflet, 'People in Wheelchairs – Hints for Helpers'.

The exact type of wheelchair you eventually choose will depend on a number of factors. Are you going to use it indoors and out? Do you want to self-propel it or be pushed? Do you want to spend a lot of money on an electric model? Most people will require a chair that's suitable for both indoor and outdoor use, which will also fold up to fit in a car, and which is comfortable.

Features which increase the comfort and ride include pneumatic tyres (which, along with the brakes, need regular checking), a good cushion and a plywood base. You can also add various accessories such as trays, and cushioned backrests.

Some decide to purchase an electric wheelchair, but they do have their disadvantages – they're very heavy, can't be folded up, require quite a lot of space, and are fairly expensive. Indoor electric wheelchairs can be provided by the DHSS, but the outdoor type have to be purchased privately.

Although the cost may be high, if you're receiving a Mobility Allowance you may be able to get help through the Motability scheme (see later in this chapter). Local authority housing departments may help with ramps and widening of doorways in the home, but you may need back-up from your general practitioner, occupational therapist and local councillor.

So, if you do decide that a wheelchair might help to increase your mobility, either permanently or just occasionally, do go and talk to some other users about their experiences and opinions on the types available, and seek the help of the professionals who can offer expert advice.

YOU AND YOUR CAR

Any M.E. sufferer who continues to drive a car ought to inform the motor licence authorities about their present medical condition. This may then involve a medical assessment on your continued 'fitness to drive'. Whether or not M.E. patients should be driving depends on each individual case, but some patients who are still driving probably should not be.

Many insurance companies also want to know about any physical or mental problems which could 'in any way impair your ability to drive', so check the small print, as you may be invalidating your policy. If in doubt most insurance companies have a medical advisor at their head office you could write to. If you do act accordingly, the insurance company will in all probability want to know what the licence authority have decided.

For those who continue to drive (in the U.K.) there are two motoring organisations specialising in the problems faced by disabled drivers (see page 203). Both the Disabled Drivers' Association and the Disabled Drivers' Motor Club can give advice on car adaptations, and membership may also help with financial concessions on car ferries, motor insurance and RAC membership.

The Mobility Advice and Vehicle Information Service (see page 208) can provide free help on mobility problems for disabled drivers, and for a fee they will give specialist individual advice on adaptations to cars. There are several centres throughout the U.K.

Motability This is a unique scheme, sponsored by the government, which is designed to help people who are already receiving a Mobility Allowance from the DHSS. The idea is to use this benefit to help with buying or leasing a car. The parents of children in receipt of a Mobility Allowance can also participate if the car is going to be used for the child's purposes. Full details can be obtained from Motability (see page 208) or from your local DHSS office.

Exemption from Road Tax This is a very useful financial benefit for anyone claiming Mobility Allowance, but the car must be used 'solely by or for the purposes of the disabled person', in the legal jargon. In other words a wife with M.E. claiming Mobility Allowance can't claim tax relief on her husband's car if he's using it all day at his work! If you receive Mobility Allowance and think you qualify, get a Vehicle Excise Duty (VED) exemption form from the DHSS. This allowance can also be claimed by some passengers who are receiving an Attendance Allowance from the DHSS.

Rates relief on a garage used to house the car of a disabled driver may be available from your local authority – phone the local rates office.

The Orange Badge parking scheme This entitles recipients with 'severe mobility problems' to various parking concessions, and is administered by the local authority. The scheme covers both disabled drivers and suitably disabled passengers, so non-drivers can apply.

To qualify you must already be receiving a Mobility Allowance, or Attendance Allowance from the DHSS, or in the legal jargon have a 'permanent and substantial disability to walk, or a very considerable difficulty in walking', something which tends to be open to a wide interpretation! A supporting letter from your GP can be of great help, as well as already being registered as disabled, but the system is being abused and it seems likely that the issuing of such concessions may in future become much stricter.

If the local authority refuses your request there is no right to any appeal, although your local councillor may help in changing their mind.

Orange Badge holders can obtain similar concessions when travelling abroad.

PUBLIC TRANSPORT

For many M.E. sufferers who've had to stop driving their cars, or never even driven, increasing reliance on what often seems to be a declining standard of public transport becomes a necessity. Fortunately, the administrators of public transport have in recent years become more aware of the needs of their disabled travellers – particularly British Rail and the airlines – and some real progress is, at last, being made.

There is also some genuine financial help available with fares on most public transport, but the level of disability to qualify varies considerably.

Local voluntary organisations are now producing a range of access guides to toilets, shops and public buildings, and RADAR (see page 210) has started a scheme of specially designed toilets for the disabled. For a fee of £2.50 you can get a special key (from RADAR) which gives automatic access to these conveniences.

British Rail charges a small fee for their disabled person's railcard which gives reduced fares for both the holder and a companion. Anyone who receives Mobility or Attendance Allowance automatically qualifies. This also now applies to those receiving the Severely Disabled Allowance, after I pointed out to British Rail that if you're deemed to be 'severely disabled' you ought to be sufficiently disabled to receive a 'disabled railcard'.

If you are severely affected by M.E., particularly if you are using a wheelchair, and want extra help during your journey do let British Rail know (in good time and to the right department) as staff can be very helpful. They produce a comprehensive leaflet, 'British Rail and Disabled Travellers', which details all the ways they will help the disabled, and whom to contact for what.

Bus travel Many local authorities give financial help by issuing concessionary fares to people who've registered as disabled. Phone the local treasurer's department for further details.

Taxis and 'dial-a-ride' schemes Some towns now operate 'dial-a-ride' schemes for disabled people, who are unable to make use of public transport. This can be of immense value for shopping trips, or just being able to get out once in a while for a social occasion. The service usually operates on a door-to-door basis. The Citizens Advice Bureau will know if there's one near you.

The London Taxicard This unique scheme is run by London Regional Transport, and enables those who qualify to only pay the first £1 in a £7 taxi fare. After £7 you pay the normal rate. You have to apply on a Taxicard application form (from the post office) and it requires your doctor's signature.

The DHSS will provide cash help with fares to hospital for those claiming low income benefits.

TAKING A HOLIDAY

Just like everyone else, people with M.E., along with their carers and relatives, need and enjoy a good holiday. However, the effort involved in getting away can be very tiring. But once you've got to the destination, a pleasant holiday in the right climate, with good accommodation and food can produce a considerable improvement.

The first thing to do is plan well ahead, and discuss with the whole family what sort of holiday seems most suitable, and where you're going to – home or abroad. Obviously, a holiday in the U.K. may be easier to get to if you're intending to go by car, and you're having to help with the driving. Alternatively, many pleasant parts of France can easily be reached using the car ferries, although this may mean the frustrations of having to hang about at odd hours, and climbing awkward stairs from the car decks. If you can't cope with stairs get in touch with the ferry operator beforehand, and they should let you use the lift. Some M.E. sufferers have invested in caravans – obviously there must be another very fit member of the party, but this is an option worth considering.

If you're particularly disabled by M.E., and especially if you have to use a wheelchair, there are many hotels which make a point of having special rooms with appropriate access and washing facilities. Again, if you have special dietary needs some hotels will be very helpful. The Disabled Drivers' Association can give further help with the sort of problems you may encounter travelling abroad.

Some M.E. sufferers make the mistake of believing that a holiday in the hot sun will improve their condition. Unfortunately this is very rarely so, and the heat often makes M.E. worse. I personally find a warm, but *not* hot, rural part of France, with clean air and good food very beneficial, avoiding the very hot summer months.

If you are going abroad do make sure that you have adequate health insurance, and check the policy carefully to make sure about exclusions for 'pre-existing medical conditions'. There are still plenty of companies who will happily provide cover for M.E. sufferers, but you may have to shop around. Going abroad should be all right, providing you don't travel 'against your doctor's advice'.

Aeroplane travel can be quite an exhausting experience, with crowded departure lounges, long walks with luggage to the planes, and the inevitable delays. If you use a wheelchair, and let the flight operator know in good time they can be immensely helpful. One friend of mine with M.E. – an occasional wheelchair user – always uses his for transit through airports. Your travel agent should be able to give you some idea on conditions in foreign airports (and hotels) if you're considering travelling abroad.

British Airways produce a useful leaflet ('Travel Wise' – for incapacitated passengers) which is available from BA Customer Services, Comet House, Heathrow Airport. This gives details about their Frequent Traveller's Card (FREMEC) for disabled passengers, and how to arrange for escorted help through arrivals/departures and getting on to the aircraft. If you're flying it may be a good idea to go to the airport the day before and stay at a hotel for the night.

Compulsory vaccinations are seldom required for most popular European holiday resorts, and the chances of picking up nasty infections are fairly remote, provided you keep to simple rules of hygiene. (For further advice, see pages 151–2.) If you get travel sickness, cinnarazine (Stugeron) is a useful drug. If you're abroad it's worth having a note of any important drugs you take already translated into the foreign tongue, just in case you lose them. The same applies for any other important medical conditions apart from M.E. The chances of finding a doctor abroad who's even heard of M.E. are going to be fairly remote.

Always try and do as much of your packing and attend to anything else that needs doing in the home several days before you're going away. Ideally, this should then leave you with a forty-eight-hour gap before you depart, in which you can rest as much as possible.

Last, don't forget about the needs of your partner or the rest of the family. If they're having to do most of the organising or driving, why not suggest an overnight stop to break the journey? Or even consider using the motorail – both here and abroad.

5. Relationships

One of the most distressing aspects of M.E. is the way it interferes with all aspects of one's personal and social life.

It can be very difficult at times maintaining your friendships, but don't ever lose the ones who are kind and understanding. There will be some who just can't comprehend what you're going through, and who will make the most stupid and insensitive suggestions about what you might try and do to get better. You're bound to find that existing friends are going to take varying attitudes towards you and your illness. The more they understand about M.E. and the way it affects you, the more likely it is that they'll remain the sort of friends you still want to see – so do explain M.E. to them.

Most sufferers will find that a whole range of sporting and social activities, which previously made life so enjoyable, now have to be abandoned or curtailed. For many sufferers this inability to participate in any form of sporting activity is a severe blow, as outside work, sports and hobbies are a very important way of meeting people and maintaining friendships. Some M.E. patients try to maintain their involvement by becoming spectators instead. It may also be possible to keep in touch by performing some sort of administrative function for the club or organisation.

This reduction of interests and social life is something which partners and carers also find difficult, and so for their sake it helps to try to have some form of 'non-active' social life together from time to time. It could just be a visit to the cinema or theatre, or a quiet meal out at a restaurant. If you really can't face the thought of going out, why not make an event out of an evening at home perhaps by hiring a good video and getting a take-away meal?

Don't ever forget about those people who are closest to you – your partner, your children and your best friends. These relationships are going to come under great strain from time to time, but these are the sort of people you're going to rely on for a great deal of support.

CARING FOR SOMEONE WHO HAS M.E.

The person who is closest to an M.E. sufferer – be it spouse, parent or child – has a very difficult job.

Suddenly, the carer finds that their family member is not the person they once were. They cannot cope, physically, as they once did, and there may be psychological problems as well such as loss of confidence and self-esteem, exaggerated mood swings and depression. Just as the sufferer is coming to terms with all sorts of problems, so may all those around him or her be experiencing similar difficulties in learning how to cope.

Caring isn't just providing physical help. Most M.E. sufferers won't need the extra sort of physical care with lifting and bathing that someone with multiple sclerosis, for example, might require. Caring involves a great deal of emotional help as well.

Neither of you can predict the eventual outcome of the disease, and this can make forward planning very difficult. M.E. patients do stand a good chance of getting better and returning to normal health and a normal way of life. Unfortunately, this can take a long time, and it's all too easy for a sufferer to give up hope when they've had M.E. for several years, and to become convinced that he or she is never going to get better.

A key part of the carer's role is not only to understand what the sufferer is putting up with, but to give hope and encouragement that recovery will take place, and keep the person in a positive frame of mind that he or she will get better. Part of this positive approach is to encourage the sufferer to look after their personal appearance, to maintain their friendships and social contacts, and pursue their work, hobbies and interests – provided they are not exceeding their capabilities, and are having the proper amount of rest.

It helps to talk about the illness. Join the M.E. Patients' Association – where at a local group meeting you'll be able to meet other people who are close to someone who's living with M.E.

M.E. sufferers will obviously have differing physical and emotional needs when it comes to receiving help from other people. Many will be the sort of individuals who haven't been used to asking for this type of assistance in the past, so it's not easy to be specific about what to do for them. Here are suggested guidelines to be followed with a wide degree of flexibility, according to each individual's needs and personality.

A FOUR-POINT PLAN TO HELP CARERS AND RELATIVES

1 Find out all you can about M.E.

One of the first practical steps that any relative or carer must take is to find out as much as possible about this illness, and the way it's affecting the sufferer.

Above all, this means listening and learning from the sufferer about how M.E. is affecting his or her life, which may mean encouraging them to express feelings about both physical and emotional difficulties – something which some people may find very hard to do, and which they haven't been used to doing in the past.

It's a good idea for both of you to go along together, on at least one occasion, to a consultation with the sufferer's general practitioner or consultant – any reasonable doctor shouldn't object to this. It's quite likely that there are questions which the sufferer may not want to ask – here the doctor may be willing to see the carer separately, but some would regard it as unethical to talk about a patient's illness without their permission. Do find out all you can about how the doctor feels the individual illness should best be managed, any drugs that are being prescribed, what sort of things cause a relapse, and whether there are any reasons for the sufferer to be seen by a specialist who's 'expert' in M.E.

It's a very natural reaction for some relatives, when an illness like M.E. has been diagnosed, to start spending vast amounts of money and time chasing an elusive 'cure'. They write to experts all over the world, and request second opinions from anyone involved with the condition. Others take a completely opposite view and almost deny that any problem exists, or that it will go away if ignored. Some are even so successful in this type of approach that they don't realise that they're doing it! If the sufferer wants to try out some 'alternative' remedies or change their diet, don't denigrate such an approach. It may help, and many patients undoubtedly feel better simply by the fact that they are now taking some management decisions about their illness.

Read all you can about the illness; it's not hard to find up-to-date medical information on M.E., and the M.E. Association can often help if you're having difficulties. Once you've got the basic facts straight in your head about how M.E. behaves as an illness, it should be a lot easier for both of you to start making the sort of essential changes in lifestyle, without which progressive recovery is unlikely.

2 Involve the whole family

Where an M.E. patient is part of a family group it's often a very good idea for all the members to get together for a sort of family conference, so that everyone can appreciate how the illness is going to affect both the sufferer and their family life.

It's an opportunity for everyone to make their feelings – positive and negative – known about any particular difficulties or anxieties, as well as reallocating some of the household and family duties. Hopefully, everyone can be flexible, and decide on practical ways of getting around any current problems. This is far better than members of the sufferer's family quietly grumbling away behind their back, and no solutions being found.

Getting children to understand the effects of M.E. on one of their parents can be a particularly difficult task. Try to explain the disease to them as honestly as possible, so they can understand why mum or dad can't do the sort of activities with, or for them, that other parents do.

Children find it very difficult to cope with a parent who has M.E. Like everyone else, some will be extremely supportive and even start to take on an adult role in the way they help about the house. Unfortunately, others will be the exact opposite, being completely unhelpful, and even isolating themselves from the sufferer and the illness.

At the age of five or six many children will want to know why mum or dad doesn't go out to work like his friends' parents, and why he or she can't come out and help with the game of football or go on a weekend camping trip. Some children will even make up fictitious occupations for you in order to avoid teasing and embarrassment at school – children can be very cruel to each other at times.

There aren't easy solutions to problems with the children, but talking to other families who are coping with M.E. might be very helpful and give you some ideas as to how some of your own problems might be tackled.

3 Get organised – find out about help that's available

Find out about all the extra sources of help and advice which are available, and might be appropriate to your particular needs and circumstances. Practical help for the disabled, and advice on social security benefits are covered comprehensively elsewhere (see pages 175–95).

Don't forget that besides friends and family, other people such as your neighbours, may be only too willing to give a bit of help – if only they were to be asked. If you are receiving help from people not closely associated with you or the sufferer, it's a great help to them if you carefully explain the nature of the illness and how it affects the sufferer. People can be quite afraid of illnesses (and sufferers of) which they don't understand, so it's important that you or the patient puts them fully in the picture. They may be quite happy to offer a bit of practical help, such as doing a bit of regular shopping each week, and you or your partner might also be able to do something for them in return, such as looking after a pet when they go on holiday.

With the loss of mobility that M.E. imposes, many M.E. sufferers will find that new friendships now come from neighbours and people living close to them, when previously they may have only known one or two people who lived in the same street.

There is a new umbrella organisation, the Association of Carers (see page 200), which now exists specifically for people who are caring or helping to look after people with disability. They act as a source of further information on a whole range of practical problems anyone acting as a carer may face. They also organise local groups where you could meet other people who are having to cope with similar feelings and experiences that you may have with M.E. It's not the sort of help that everyone requires, but it's there should you need it.

4 Self-help for the carer

It's all too easy, when caring for somebody else, to start putting your own interests and life into second place. After all, you're trying to perform a kind of balancing act between your own needs, the rest of the family, and caring for your partner. It can become easy to start neglecting your own health, both physical and emotional, and it's no use falling ill as well, when you've become the central pillar to family life. If you find yourself getting depressed, do go and seek help from your general practitioner, or try to arrange for a counselling session. And if you've got any physical symptoms, don't neglect them – do go and get them sorted out.

You'll also have a lot of personal feelings about the way M.E. is affecting both your lives; some will be positive, but many will be negative and upsetting. You'll probably start to get fed up at times (just like the sufferer) about the restrictions M.E. is placing on your life. You may start to feel despondent when the sufferer doesn't seem to be making any real progress, or some new treatment isn't having any effect.

All this is a very natural reaction. There aren't any *easy* solutions, but whatever feelings you do have about either the sufferer, or the M.E., try not to bottle them up. If you don't find it easy to discuss them with the sufferer, it can help a lot to talk to a close friend or relative, or the partner of another M.E. sufferer whom you may have met at a local group meeting. Such a third party may even be able to intervene and help defuse a family crisis by tactfully putting your point of view about a particular issue.

Unfortunately, there may be times when the relationship between you and the sufferer comes under great stress, even crisis. If you find it very difficult dealing with frustrations or putting your feelings into words, try writing them down. It's something of a last resort, but just occasionally it can be very effective to relieve the pressure.

A variety of pressures may build up: health, personal and financial worries. It can be very helpful to talk things over with someone completely detached from the family. This might be a social worker, a sympathetic general practitioner, or even a professional or volunteer counsellor. (The British Association of Counselling trains such people – see page 200.)

Although you may find that for much of the time you're having to put your interests, and even your work, into second place it's terribly important not to abandon them altogether.

It's unusual for any M.E. sufferer to actually require full-time physical help throughout the day, so giving up work for that reason isn't usually necessary. However, when a wife with small children develops M.E. (especially if they're of pre-school age) the husband may well have to make some very major decisions regarding his own employment, especially if he spends a large amount of time away from home. Alternatively, if the bread-winner has had to give up work due to M.E., it may be the carer who's now got to consider going out to work, for purely financial reasons and on top of all the other responsibilities. Making the correct decisions in such circumstances is not easy, so do try and talk to other people who've had to make similar decisions before finally making up your mind.

If you're already working and happy in what you're doing, and there are no practical problems at home, there are good reasons for you to continue. It gives you respite from each other, and the opportunity to continue with outside friendships and social life. Also, do try not to give up hobbies and interests, even though there may be practical difficulties, or activities which you can no longer do together any more.

Don't feel guilty about going out on your own once or twice a week to an evening class, or a game of sport with some friends, even though your partner isn't well enough to come. It is important, at the same time, to try and develop some new interests and hobbies which you can do together. This might be swimming, a gentle walk in the countryside, or a trip out to a meal or the cinema if your partner feels well enough.

SEXUAL RELATIONSHIPS AND M.E.

Sexual feelings are a natural and essential part of any caring relationship, especially in the age group affected by M.E. In fact, sex may be one of the few pleasurable physical activities that sufferers still feel they can enjoy.

It's hardly surprising that many M.E. patients experience sexual problems at some time during their illness, with, probably, both physical and emotional factors interacting. Any sufferer who is going through a bad patch may withdraw emotionally from those around him. When this happens, the partner may feel rejected, so he or she loses interest in sexual activity as well. Some M.E. patients may also develop a negative body image, no longer seeing themselves attractive to their partner, and in such cases experienced psychosexual counselling can be very helpful.

Patients who have become anxious or depressed because of the illness, especially when they are taking some of the prescribed drugs, will find this often causes a further dampening down of sexual feelings. Normal sexual arousal stimulates nerves which help open up the tiny blood vessels in the penis to allow an erection to take place. Any anxiety will dampen down this nervous activity, and if the male partner fails on one occasion to achieve an erection, subsequent anxiety about a repetition may prevent him achieving an erection on the next occasion. Male impotence isn't a part of the physical disease process in M.E. When it does occur, emotional factors are probably much more significant.

For some patients, the physical problems associated with M.E. may make sex no longer an appealing activity. Pain in the muscles and joints may severely limit capabilities, and of course, sexual intercourse does involve the expenditure of a large amount of energy in a very short space of time. Intimacy doesn't have to end in intercourse, so foreplay, caressing and touching can be equally satisfying, as an alternative to 'active sex', if the energy just isn't there.

If pain in the muscles, joints or back is a significant factor in reducing sexual pleasure, try taking a warm bath before going to bed, and consider taking an aspirin or other anti-inflammatory drug a couple of hours before. Back pain can be eased by placing a pillow under the lower back of the partner in the passive position. Don't be afraid to explore new positions which you may find more comfortable. Get a 'guide book' if you're not quite sure what to do! A man with M.E. will use much less energy if he lies underneath, and the wife becomes the active partner. Alternatively, lying side-by-side may be more comfortable.

Sex can also be therapeutic. Arthritis sufferers sometimes report pain relief following orgasm, which is thought to be due to the release from the brain of chemicals known as endorphins, which are like the body's self-produced morphine.

If you are experiencing sexual difficulties, do get help. Some GPs are excellent, as in other aspects of M.E., but others don't have a clue when it comes to sexual problems, and are just as embarrassed as their patients. If your GP doesn't seem the right person to approach, then the local family planning clinic or marriage guidance council will point you in the right direction. The British Association of Counselling have counsellors available and SPOD (Sexual and Personal Relationships of People with a Disability) can also provide advice and help (see page 212).

PART 3
LEARNING TO LIVE WITH M.E.

1. Three Case Histories

LOOKING AFTER A YOUNG CHILD WHO HAS M.E.
by Rachael Glover's mother

At eight years of age my daughter Rachael was an outgoing, active and very cheerful child, who enjoyed ballet lessons, gymnastics and long country walks. At the crack of dawn she'd be up, singing around the house, and generally driving us all to distraction with her 'get up and go'. She loved school, and couldn't wait to get there each morning. She even wanted to go at the weekends! Alas, I didn't realise how precious a time it was for us, and I now look back on those eight short years as being Rachael's childhood. For she was then struck down, quite dramatically, with what our GP thought was glandular fever.

Rachael had swollen glands, a temperature and an ulcerated sore throat. She was racked with pain all over her body, and this continued for several weeks. However, all the blood tests came back as normal, so we were told to get her back to school as soon as possible.

As time went on her symptoms didn't seem to improve, so I asked for a referral to the local hospital. The consultant agreed with our GP's opinion and felt she would be fully better within three months, and to continue going to school. She went back, but was too weary to take part in the general activities, preferring to sit in a quiet corner. The teachers were convinced that she'd become used to being at home, and wouldn't accept my doubts and fears concerning her non-recovery.

Rachael would only be in school for a couple of days before collapsing with the return of all her previous symptoms. Even when she did manage to go she was never totally well, and this continued for two years. Daily living was never ever to be the same again for any of the family. We attempted to go on one of our favourite walks one Sunday, when she appeared to be a little brighter, but after only 300 yards she collapsed and had to be carried home. So started the awful lethargy which has since dominated her life.

One day, looking through the family snapshots, trying to amuse her, I was shocked to realise the drastic change which had occurred. Gone were the lovely rosy cheeks and bright eyes, only to be replaced by a deathly pallor and dark circles under the eyes. I took her back to the hospital where she had every conceivable blood test they could do, but in the end the advice was that she should pull herself together, and stop thinking of herself as being an invalid.

We returned to our GP, and this time asked for a second opinion at Great Ormond Street children's hospital, in London. There we were told that, yes, Rachael was poorly, but they didn't actually know what was the cause. The consultant said he'd come across children like this before, and that after a time they always made a recovery, but he didn't know what ailed them. He continued to see Rachael on a regular basis, and fully backed us up with, for example, countless letters to the school, and most important of all gave us lots of moral support. However, other doctors and teachers involved with Rachael continued to maintain that there was nothing much wrong with her.

As so often happens when one has almost given up hope, I turned on the radio one evening and found myself listening to

Dr Shepherd talking about M.E. It hit me that this was exactly what Rachael was suffering from. I duly got in touch with the M.E. Association, and was put in touch with another doctor who was experienced in M.E. After listening to our story, examining Rachael, and further blood tests, it turned out that Rachael had a positive test for enterovirus in the blood, strongly supporting the diagnosis of M.E. The medical advice was that there was no 'cure', but with rest – both physical and mental – she would eventually get over it. We felt a great relief that, at last, we'd got a diagnosis of what was wrong.

By now Rachael was starting to require a wheelchair to go any distance, and by the time of her last Christmas at junior school it was necessary to push her to the local church for the carol concert.

There were times of despair and one particularly awful night she said: 'Mummy, it would be kinder to gas me, than to let me suffer like this any longer.' I was shocked and so very sad for her. We had a little weep together, but I felt so angry that my child was having to suffer for so long in this way.

In the midst of all this the school decided to threaten us with prosecution for Rachael's constant non-attendance. This resulted in a meeting with the Chief Education Officer to try and sort out the mounting difficulties concerning Rachael's education, or rather the lack of it. At last we seemed to have someone who was totally on our side. Soon after the meeting a letter arrived from the school, not quite an apology, but near enough, plus a pile of kind letters from all the children in Rachael's class.

It was arranged for us to have the services of a home tutor, and the authority decided that Rachael should be 'statemented'. We'd never heard of this procedure before, so I contacted the group leader of CASE (Campaign for the Advancement of State Education), as well as the Advisory Centre for Education (see page 199) and received a lengthy reply – all very much in favour of the statementing procedure. Statementing is basically a legal term connected with the English 1981 Education Act. It's a means of assessing the educational requirements of a sick or disabled child. It highlights the needs or support the child requires, be it a home tutor, flexible school hours, tutor support whilst in school lessons, provision of wheelchairs and ramps, etc. It outlines virtually everything the child needs within the school environment.

The process involves meetings between medical representatives, teachers, a child psychologist from the education department, along with the parents. Written evidence can also be submitted. If the parents disagree with the findings there are procedures available to have decisions changed. When it's been decided exactly what help is required a 'statement' is then prepared. When everyone is fully satisfied with this final statement it's placed with the local authority, who must carry out all the recommendations, and make any necessary funds available. If the school doesn't comply with any of the required tasks the authority can make it do so. In essence, it's well worth having, and so far it's certainly been of great help to us.

A home tutor was provisionally allocated to Rachael for five hours a week. This was more than enough, as she was rarely well enough for more. The teacher was fully aware of the problems created by M.E., and on the days when Rachael was well enough they'd read stories, and sometimes play a board game. Unfortunately, they rarely managed to accomplish much real work as Rachael's concentration was so low. However, it was nice for Rachael to have this type of company and help – a lady who could be trusted not to push her beyond her limitations. It also gave me the first chance in many months to have an hour or so to myself.

Children with M.E. do require a great deal of help and support when trying to return to school. Your child, like mine, may have been extremely bright and able prior to M.E., but now with concentration difficulties and muscle fatigue to contend with, they may find themselves increasingly forced into the situation where they need a statement in order to receive the requisite help.

In September 1987 Rachael joined her new secondary school, although she didn't actually make her first appearance until February 1988. The school was our choice, even before it became obvious that she now had very specific needs. It's well known in the area for its high standards of education, coupled with a strong belief in caring for less fortunate pupils, who find the staff helpful and sympathetic to their needs. The school has ramps, a lift and other adaptations for pupils with disabilities. At present there are six children who need these aids. Disabled children are encouraged to take part in all aspects of school life wherever possible, but if, like Rachael, rest is the name of the game, they go to great lengths to make sure that they don't overdo things.

By Christmas 1987, Rachael had been ill for four years. She hadn't yet met her classmates, but the children sent her a massive pile of beautifully written letters, jokes and stories. They said that the teacher and matron had often talked about her, so they felt they already knew Rachael, and looked forward to the day when she'd be well enough to join them. Girls had already volunteered to push her chair and be helpers. Needless to say this was all received with much joy, and she started to look forward to being well enough to be able to go next term.

As her health gradually improved I left it entirely up to Rachael to decide when to start her first day. In January she proudly hung up her new school uniform on the wardrobe door, and began to collect her pens and equipment together for the big day. We had a few false starts, but by mid-February she felt well enough to go for one lesson per day. I took her to school by car, and she was pushed in her wheelchair to meet the new class-mates.

After that one short visit she was exhausted, and lay on the settee for the rest of the day. In the first week she only managed the one lesson, but after that she gradually built things up, until she was actually staying for school lunches with her new-found friends – always the same baked beans and chips, but who cares! – then home to rest. Suddenly she was a different girl, starting to feel a bit better day by day, and taking an interest in life again.

For me, this had been a very difficult time, having to stand back and watch her first few tentative steps, wanting to stop her from doing too much, but realising how important it was for her to learn for herself. It wasn't long before she'd actually accomplished three weeks of full-time schooling. There was nothing stopping her now. I'd hold my breath and clamp my lips firmly shut as she played in the garden with her friends, running to and fro. However, by bedtime one evening, the results of all this new activity were beginning to show. After a restless night she awoke once again with swollen glands, and feeling very low. I must say, though, she didn't get as unwell as I'd feared, and she didn't slip back too far. Recovering from M.E. can be two steps forward and one step back. Her level of activity – both physical and mental – still obviously at a much reduced level, but a year earlier I had truly believed that my daughter had no future at all.

Her teachers have given her wonderful reports: 'keen, willing to work and a pleasure to teach' are all music to my ears. She still has to have a home tutor to sit with her for some lessons, as well as help from a welfare assistant during craft lessons. And instead of P.E., she spends time with the matron doing gentle exercises.

Rachael is now twelve-and-a-half years old, and is still painfully thin and frail. She gets tired very quickly, and has to rely heavily on her wheelchair to get around outside the house. The local school for the handicapped have a warm pool, and they've kindly agreed to let Rachael use it for half an hour each week. She just goes and lies in the water, and the physiotherapist gives her some gentle exercises in the pool. She is getting better, improving slowly day by day, and one day I'm sure that all of this will just be a painful memory.

I don't think that children of Rachael's age can ever come to terms with an illness of this magnitude – neither can many adults. She accepts that she has a strange disease, and is heartily sick and tired of it, but she still refuses to take any interest in it. The only time she'll put herself out to discuss M.E. is if she hears of another child going through black days with it, and then she tries to help them feel a bit better. She no longer plans ahead; she just says she'll see how she feels on the day before deciding what to do. She used to cry a lot, but now she tries to laugh things off by saying that it's 'only the bugs' which are bothering her. Until quite recently she didn't like to talk about her future aspirations, but now she talks about doing 'something with computers', so she's obviously feeling much more confident about the future.

The financial pressures on the family have been quite considerable during the course of Rachael's illness, especially at a time when I'd planned to return to full-time employment again. This I had to forgo in order to be at home to look after Rachael. In view of her quite severe disability we applied for both an

Attendance Allowance and a Mobility Allowance. Since then, like so many others, we've had to endure the full bureaucratic nightmare of the DHSS system. The examining doctor for Rachael's Mobility Allowance wrote that she fulfilled the requirements, as the exertion required to walk exacerbated her illness. However, it then came as a shock to find this had been turned down by the authorities, who make the final decision. We decided to appeal, but the next doctor decided she was perfectly able to walk the required distance. The next stage is an appeal to the tribunal, but when you're physically and mentally worn down by caring for someone the last thing you want (or are capable of) is fighting for benefits. I've found a welfare rights worker, attached to the Benefits Unit of the town hall. They help prepare your case, and will even attend the tribunal with you.

As for the family, Rachael's illness has taken its toll on us all. Our youngest daughter, Emma, just eleven, has missed out more than anyone else on holidays, trips out, picnics, etc. Most of the time she's been uncomplaining, but just occasionally she would get bitterly upset and jealous about the disproportionate amount of attention Rachael was getting. Fortunately I'm now in a position to be able to spend more time with Emma, and am trying to mend the damage. But, just like Rachael, these precious years can never be replaced. It's not been quite the same for my sons, and Ben, who's now seventeen, is happy with his own friends away at college.

M.E. has taught us many things: first and foremost to take each day as it comes. If your child can't eat, sleep or whatever, don't worry – maybe they will tomorrow. When, as undoubtedly they will, your child begins to start taking the first tentative steps back to normal life, learn to stand back, as they've now got to find their own level of activity, and learn to have control over their own lives again.

Ignorance of this disease has only made Rachael's suffering worse, and I think the illness has lasted longer as a result. If only I'd known at the beginning what I know now, I think I could have handled things much more easily. Complete bed rest from the onset would, I believe, have significantly aided her recovery.

Believe, really believe, deep in your heart, that your own

child can and will get better from M.E. It happens slowly but surely – just you wait and see.

CHILDREN WITH M.E.: AUTHOR'S NOTE

M.E. is not an illness which often affects young children. When it does occur, the symptoms are generally similar to those seen in adults, although there are some characteristic features, which include:

- Sleep pattern disturbances which can be very pronounced, with the child sleeping by day and then awake at night. Nightmares and irritability frequently accompany this problem.
- Some boys develop difficulties with passing urine.
- These children may lose a significant amount of weight and become very weak.

Obtaining a diagnosis is often a far more frustrating process than for adults, as some paediatricians do not recognise M.E. A clumsy management strategy is then adopted – the child is forced to return to full-time schooling along with lots of physical exercise (the 'in at the deep end' approach) and this results in a further deterioration in both physical and emotional symptoms.

The broad principles of management are the same as for adults, taking into account the fact that children obviously have their own emotional, practical and educational problems. Unfortunately, in some cases a child develops a clinging dependency on the parents, who in turn become over-protective and unduly cautious about tackling any of the negative aspects of this illness. The child starts to stagnate, becoming socially isolated, and experiences very little in the way of constructive mental stimulation. Even though the physical side of the illness may be improving, they have become trapped by the psychological aspects of M.E.

If this circle can be broken in a firm but fair manner many of these children can turn the corner and start to make a significant degree of recovery. They require a lot of encouragement to start joining in with all aspects of family life, even if this means taking away the TV in their bedroom, and accepting that they will drop some dishes if they help with the washing-up!

Planning a return to school is the most difficult aspect of recovery. This must be managed using a multidisciplinary approach involving the family doctor, education department, home tutor and possibly an educational psychologist. Careful advance planning should include arranging transport, avoiding any exam pressures and initially being flexible about the time spent at school. The statement procedure, described in the case history, is very useful here.

It is not easy finding specialist doctors interested and experienced in dealing with children who have M.E. This is important, because sometimes the only way of helping such a child is to admit them to hospital for a short period, where a full assessment of physical and emotional symptoms can be made, and a co-ordinated rehabilitation programme planned. The good news is that children do recover from M.E., but it may be the psychological part of the illness which is holding them back.

PREGNANCY AND M.E.
by Frances H. Woodward

I had been suffering from M.E. for two and a half years before we decided to have a baby. It was a very difficult decision to make because, at that time, my 'vertical hours' averaged only about five or six a day. My best time was, and still is, in the mornings. I would get up and potter around doing small jobs but by early afternoon I would start to fade away and for the rest of the time I was in bed. So my daily routine was not exactly congenial to having a baby.

One factor which encouraged us was that my condition was gradually improving. I'd had quite a dramatic start to my illness when, in March 1982, I had viral meningitis. I was in hospital for a week, and then in bed at home for several weeks. During the following months I suffered extreme fatigue: sometimes brushing my teeth was all I could manage before having to go back to bed. My doctor said that it was a slow recovery from meningitis, but I knew there was something else wrong with me. I was experiencing more and more symptoms: muscle pain, back and neck pains, head pressure, difficulty in walking and extreme fatigue. After almost a year I was eventually sent to a neurologist and he diagnosed benign myalgic encephalomyelitis. I couldn't believe there was an illness with such a long name and thought I would never remember it! I was, in fact, greatly relieved that what I was feeling had a name.

I immediately joined the M.E. Association and discovered the importance of rest and sleep. Instead of trying to push myself to do things, I established a new daily routine. I would get up in the mornings, at first for only one or two hours and then return to bed. Gradually, over the next year or so, I increased those vertical hours to five or six.

My husband and I had always wanted children and were anxious that this debilitating disease might prevent it. My GP and the specialist had suggested it would not be a good idea. However, in May 1984, we asked the advice of Dr Smith, the M.E. Association Medical Advisor. His advice was what we wanted to hear. If we really wanted children then life without them may make us unhappy and discontent. It was better to go ahead, being fully aware of the problems and with the provision of plenty of help.

When my pregnancy was confirmed, in January 1985, I really became very anxious about whether our decision had been wise. I wrote to Dr Smith for reassurance and also to another M.E. sufferer who had had a baby. Her letter boosted my morale as she was coping well and was, in fact, expecting her second child.

My first visit to the hospital was interesting because, at that time, little was known about M.E. The nurses and midwives were all interested to know how the disease affected me, were sympathetic in their manner and admired our decision to battle against the odds and have a baby. The gynaecologist had little experience of M.E. but suspected that I would cope all right with the first stage of labour but might have a problem in the second stage and be incapable of pushing. As I was thirty-seven, he recommended an amniocentesis which I had at sixteen weeks. My stomach was sore and uncomfortable for a week afterwards and I found it difficult to stand upright. Presumably this was because with M.E. the muscles are particularly tender and take longer to recover. Anyway, three weeks later the results came through as clear, so all was well.

I think having M.E. prepared me quite well for the aches and pains of pregnancy. In fact, the slight and temporary discomfort seemed mild compared to the long-term and severe pain and fatigue of M.E. I was used to resting and pacing myself – other people have to learn to do that while pregnant. Gradually, however, over the nine months, my M.E. symptoms eased. The acute pains I suffered in my neck, head, back and arms seemed to be duller but the major relief I had was the fading of that awful 'ill' feeling. My head cleared, and although I still get pressure in my head, that mental numbness which was constantly with me disappeared. I felt almost part of the real world; almost a real person instead of a zombie!

I must explain here that all during my pregnancy I was having acupuncture. I had started a course of treatment about three months before I became pregnant, in an anxious attempt to do something positive to help myself. It is difficult to judge which made me feel better – pregnancy or acupuncture – but I am inclined to attribute the growing feeling of well being to pregnancy and the more specific relief of things such as heart palpitations and nerve pains to acupuncture. These two problems were very severe before I started acupuncture and were starting to decline before I became pregnant. Even though I am no longer having acupuncture, they have never returned with such severity.

During the later weeks of pregnancy we discussed with the consultant the possibility of a Caesarean if labour became too much for me. General anaesthetic can worsen M.E. symptoms so it was decided that an epidural Caesarean would be our best option.

I thoroughly enjoyed my pregnancy. Not only was I relieved of some of my symptoms but I developed a sense of purpose. Previously I had felt worthless, now I had something to live for.

In August 1985, our daughter Anna was born. As the consultant predicted, I could cope with the first stage of labour, but by the second stage I was completely exhausted. I had no urge to push and no strength to push either. It was decided to use forceps. Anna was very solid (8½ lb) and needed tremendous tugging to get her into the world – an experience I would not want to endure again!

The nurses on the ward were marvellous. I had been in labour for seventeen hours and was totally exhausted. I could not walk for about twenty-four hours and during that time they brought me bed pans and gave me bed baths. When Anna cried a nurse would give her to me to feed and then return her to her cot to save me the effort. My arms were too weak to hold her so I fed her lying down. At night the babies were taken to the nursery and mothers were woken to go and feed their babies there. I did not have to do that. A nurse would bring Anna to me, return to change sides and then return again to take her back to the nursery. This was such a help to me, and whenever I expressed my appreciation they merely said that's what they were there for. I was touched by their kindness and regard for my problems. One sister even stayed on duty late one night in order to show my husband how to change a nappy and bath the baby. She had realised that he would be doing much of the caring when we got home, and took it upon herself to teach him. We really appreciated her concern.

I stayed in hospital for six days after the birth before I felt strong enough to go home. My husband took the first week off work and then my mother came for a week so it was a little while before I had to cope on my own.

We had decided that my limited energy should be concentrated on Anna and looking after her. We employed a cleaner to do the housework and a child minder to have Anna for two afternoons or whenever I needed a rest. We installed such labour saving devices as a microwave, a tumble drier and a dishwasher. I used disposable nappies to save time and effort. I could not have coped with carrying a nappy bucket, let alone washing and drying them. I find hanging clothes on the line difficult and still only put them out if it's a perfect day. There's nothing worse than having the effort of bringing clothes in, because of rain, before your arms have recovered from putting them out. If I am having a bad day or there is hint of rain I use the tumble drier.

I found breast feeding worked well for me. Those who prefer to bottle feed have the advantage that other people can help – especially at night. However, I enjoyed breast feeding and found it very relaxing. My arms were weak and my back prone to spasm, so I lay down to feed Anna, which was restful for me and cosy and comfortable for us both.

To save my arms I would lift Anna and then sit down so her weight was supported on my lap. If she needed cuddling at length I would wear a baby carrier. I bought a second-hand carry cot which was left permanently in the car, so that I only had Anna to carry in and out – not a carry cot as well. To save my back and leg muscles I had two sets of changing equipment, one upstairs and one downstairs, with the mat at table height to save bending. I only ever tried to do one task a day, apart from caring for Anna. I would see a friend, or do a little shopping, or go to the clinic, all on different days.

My husband helped with the more strenuous daily tasks. He would empty the nappy bucket (used for disposables), put out or bring in washing, do ironing, empty the dishwasher, push the shopping trolley and often cook the meal. His main daily task was bathing Anna. I found it impossible to bend forward and hold her, so bath time was his time.

Motherhood with M.E. would be virtually impossible without a sensitive and willing partner. My husband has been indispensable in the caring for Anna. As well as all the daily tasks he helps with, every Saturday and Sunday afternoon he takes over completely while I go to bed and rest.

Although having a baby is hard work and often very tiring, the rewards far outweigh the difficulties. Anna has brought joy to our lives. She has given me an aim in life and stopped me focusing my attention on myself. When I'm in pain or feeling down, her smile uplifts me and a cuddle makes it all worthwhile.

We are so glad that we risked the consequences of having a baby. Not all people with M.E. have experienced the relief of symptoms during pregnancy, but I'm sure they will all agree that life with a baby is a reward to be treasured.

M.E. AND THE SINGLE PERSON
by 'Sue'

Perhaps the first thing to say is that coping with M.E., whatever your circumstances – alone, with a partner, with children or other dependants – is made a good deal easier once a diagnosis has been made, especially if one's nearest and dearest can then understand what is happening and are able to be supportive. It cannot be stressed enough, to anyone reading this who may have M.E., or who knows someone who may have it: seek out a consultant and get a diagnosis made. To an M.E. sufferer it makes a world of difference just knowing what the matter is. It means that your self-esteem doesn't take such a knock, and that you don't go making things worse. No more feeling 'I should be able to do this so easily. Why can't I?', and no more pushing beyond personal limits. One can then take account of the illness in practical planning from day to day. So much of the secret of dealing with M.E. is illness management – but first you have to know the beast you're dealing with.

I write as someone who has had the syndrome for the best part of twenty-five years. It started in my teens, and I am forty now. I have only known what is wrong with me for three of those years. My illness has followed a chronic relapsing/remitting course, with about five prolonged, major outbreaks and never quite feeling 'well' in between-times. For years, I've alternated between saying to myself, 'Oh, this is just how I am. Not much stamina. Always tired. Often ill,' and asking, 'Do other people ever feel like this, and so often? Surely there must be something fundamentally wrong with me?' Now I know!

For part of my twenty-five 'M.E. years' I was married. So, in writing about coping with M.E. now, as a person who lives on her own, I can also look back and compare lifestyles. Such comparisons are difficult, however, because the major difference between previous years and now is not between being married and being single, but between not knowing and knowing what is wrong. My basic message would be that coping with M.E. has its good and bad, its difficult and easier bits, irrespective of your personal situation. The great divide lies between before and after diagnosis.

Once that diagnosis has been made, the next hurdle is acceptance, and learning to live within your limitations. Glibly said. At first, and perhaps for some time, there will be trial and error. You have to find out what you can do, and when to stop, to prevent a relapse. One way in which living alone can be a real boon, is that it's so much easier to leave tasks half-done, to be flexible, and alter a set routine, if you don't have a family to look after, or anyone else to take daily account of. Conversely, of course, there is no one there to help either. Shopping, cooking, cleaning, washing, and all the other household chores have to be managed, spaced out between periods of rest. Forward-planning has to be done with military precision.

If someone with M.E. lives alone there are several things that make life a bit easier. First, friends can be persuaded to form a rota to do basic tasks. If that is difficult to organise, or if a sufferer prefers to seek out voluntary help on a less personal basis, then most towns have a Council for Voluntary Service, and some have a university or a polytechnic where students may have formed a 'caring group'. Or use your local church if you have one. A phone call to any of these places can produce a team of helpers. The key is not to be afraid to ask for help, not to be deterred by apparent rebuffs, and to keep on asking until you do succeed.

For shopping, be on the look-out for firms that will deliver, and large stores that operate special bus services, often door-to-door. Some health-food stores in particular offer delivery services. Ask around, and don't hesitate to make your special needs clear. You may find – especially with a health-food store – that many customers have problems with carrying their supplies, and just one query can trigger the start of a delivery service. Also, find out if your area operates a dial-a-ride system for the disabled. Contact the Disability Unit of the council, the Passenger Transport Authority and/or social services. If there is nothing – ask for one! It can help, not just with shopping, but with any trips that you have to make.

To take the best advantage of bulk-shopping a small freezer is invaluable for single sufferers. I find it is also useful for 'bulk cooking' if and when I feel like it (and a food processor is also a boon). And I always make sure that, along with a well-stocked freezer, plenty of fresh fruit and vegetables, and all the healthy, yeast-free foods, I also have convenience foods and a range of items that are easy to prepare. Then I am ready for the bad days, because I know that however careful I am, there will be relapses.

If, like me, you have a lot of muscle problems, or arthritis, or heart problems; or if you just have the whole syndrome badly, and are more often 'flat out' than not, then do not hesitate to apply for a home help too. I have one who just does the vacuum-cleaning. The rest I can manage without too much damage, but vacuuming takes me ages, is very painful, and finishes me off afterwards, for days. In other words: choose carefully what you can do without ill effect, and follow up all channels of possible help for what you can't do. Contact with the home help section of your nearest social services office is also likely to produce an initial visit from a social worker, along with the home help organiser. This can be a helpful contact to have in reserve for if the going gets really rough and extra help (meals-on-wheels, household aids and so on) is needed.

Once you have your basic routine and regular sources of help all sorted out, it is also good to work out, *in advance*, ways of coping with times of crisis – when you feel so ill you think you're dying, and can't do a thing for yourself. If you can, get yourself an emergency 'back-up team', using the kinds of resources and techniques described above: friends, various volunteers, home help, social services. Make it clear to these people in advance what your requirements will be if you do have a long period of bad relapse: meals cooked, washing done, all the shopping, and so on. Divide out the tasks, so that people are prepared to take on whatever they can best cope with. Get it all sorted out when you are having a reasonably good patch, and so have your 'emergency services' at the ready for when you are most decidedly not. Just the knowledge that you have such a team of people to call on can be a great security blanket. Likewise, being on the telephone is a great comfort, especially with an extension by the bed. If you can't afford the luxury of a telephone, investigate whether your local council offers financial help with a phone for those in special need.

If you feel too ill to remain at home during a relapse, a referral from your GP to a local consultant and a hospital admission for short-term bed rest and nursing can be invaluable. If that can't be achieved, then another possibility to consider is going on a 'retreat', if necessary using the Ambulance Service to get there and back! Some religious orders offer board and lodging irrespective of one's beliefs or denomination. It can be a good way of obtaining rest and being looked after, if friends or relations can't produce a short-term place to stay, and if there is no hospital bed in time of crisis. Ideally, however, a good back-up team will make it possible to remain at home even during the worst of a relapse.

For M.E. sufferers living alone, perhaps the worst problems actually start when both the routine mechanics of life and crisis management have been sorted out. All too often the illness leaves one with just enough energy to cope with basic survival, and no more. But what of work, social life and hobbies? What indeed!

My current bout of M.E. has been my worst ever: really quite bad for about six years, though I am now, slowly, getting better. I have had to stop work (I get Invalidity Benefit) and have now reconciled myself to not being able to do my old job again. It is too hectic, too physically, emotionally and mentally demanding. Work has always been a major part of my life and a large chunk of my identity, and not being able to continue has been a considerable loss. And yet, changing my perspective in this regard, looking at new ways in which I can value myself and enjoy being alive, without such a work-centred existence has been a very productive experience. Many M.E. sufferers have a 'work-centred' outlook – we are often busy, energetic kinds of people.

Those of us who live on our own are perhaps even more likely to put a lot into our work. However, if stopped in our tracks by M.E. we are also the lucky ones, because we have an opportunity to try to reorientate ourselves without the added worry of letting our families down. We can apply for benefit, and, after a period of adjustment, can come to enjoy a more balanced lifestyle. Perhaps, eventually, we can find a less demanding job, if well enough. I am not saying that giving up on work is an easy process. It requires a lot of effort to change a lifetime's habit. But it can be a process that offers its own rewards – and professional help is obtainable if necessary to assist in making the adjustment. (Ask your GP for a referral to a psychologist; seek out local counselling services, again via your GP; or, if that fails, your local Community Health Council.)

If one can continue at work, then it is essential to be quite up-front about what is going on. If people know about the M.E. many will understand, make allowances, and be supportive. Job-sharing, going temporarily part-time, working from home, can all be discussed as possible solutions to the difficulties presented by the illness. But first, before they can help, people have to know what it is they are dealing with.

And then what of the rest of life? For those of us who have the illness badly that has to be very restricted too. Often the M.E. sufferer who is a little less ill, and so able to carry on working, is too exhausted to do anything else. There is no energy left for friends, going out: all the things that normally get taken for granted, and that make it good to be alive. And, all too easily, friendships fall away, people lose touch, and the sufferer living on his/her own becomes increasingly isolated. So, what to do?

Once again, it helps to be well-organised and not backward in announcing one's needs loud and clear. I try to take the initiative most of the time in organising visits to and from friends, and other social events, so that I have control of when I do things, and can plan surrounding time accordingly. I discourage chance visits because I find I have to keep a strict control on the energy I put out each day. One unexpected caller can drain resources, easily overload a day, and set me back, for several days. However, I find that it is sometimes essential to remind myself that having control over my contact with others is how I want it to be. The temptation can be to 'bleat' if people, out of consideration for my needs, do not take the initiative to contact me! One can't have it both ways!

Despite all the problems, the illness can have a positive effect on social life. It doesn't just illustrate who friends really are, but also forces one to reassess the bases of friendships – what one values friends for and vice versa. Friends can play an important part, too, in broadening out a sufferer's life beyond the confines of M.E. This is particularly essential for the sufferer living alone. Often, I think, this is an easier role for friends to play than asking them to be a sympathetic ear about the illness itself. For sufferers on their own it is perhaps particularly difficult to share the various facets of the illness with others, because so few people see us at our worst. Most, therefore, will not know what the whole syndrome is really like. (At our worst we are often stuck behind closed doors, and usually alone.) So, for the sufferer alone, perhaps the best people to turn to to discuss the illness are other sufferers in similar circumstances. The 'Singles' Group run by those members of the M.E. Association who are living alone can be of particular help here.

Useful though friends and acquaintances can be, the bedrock of being able to deal with the illness successfully has to lie inside yourself. It is necessary, if possible, to develop a sense of self-value and enjoyment of your own company, of small details, the daily minutiae of life, that can be savoured on your own: having a few plants and watching them grow; a beautiful picture to look at; a tree outside, and so on. I suppose it is a bit like holding an individual glass bead up to the light, turning and turning it, and watching how the light changes, rather than trying to string whole necklaces together, one after the other. It *is* possible to arrive at a whole new perspective on life and how to relish it; learning how to live totally in the present, moment by moment, giving all that one has (however much or little) to whatever one is doing. To live fully and completely in the present is an opportunity that doesn't come at all in most people's lives and is a real gift. For those of us who are on our own this 'gift' can also be fairly easy to obtain. Once we have our basic routine established, together with appropriate back-up for times of crisis, we can afford, within that framework, to savour the freedom that being ill can bestow, get the most out of little things, without the pressure of also having to respond to others' needs on a day-to-day basis. It is remembering this that most sustains me at all those other times, when I feel very alone, berate the restrictions of being ill, and wish there was someone there to talk to, get me a meal, or sympathise over the pain.

What also keeps me going is 'breaking out' occasionally. A person alone lacks people to sound-off to about the illness. A lot of the time he or she simply has to keep going because there is no one else there to take over. Occasionally having a good cry does wonders for pent-up frustration, grief, anger and loss – and to get these emotions out can only be good for enhancing the prospects of long-term recovery. Likewise, giving yourself a treat can help – even if that treat is detrimental in the short term and causes a temporary flare-up of symptoms. Sometimes it is good simply to 'live' and take the consequences of any flare-up that comes after. In such ways it is possible to overcome some of the feelings of loss, sadness and frustration caused by M.E.

So far I have talked of loss in conjunction with not being able to work, and not being able to pursue an active social life. There is one other important area to look at: the effect M.E. has on a person's ability to sustain a close, sexual relationship.

Some of us 'aloners' may have a sexual relationship with a partner, although we may not actually share a house. The amount of energy and effort needed if two people are to sustain a close, loving sexual relationship whilst living apart can become, at worst, prohibitive and, at best, a great source of stress, if one partner develops M.E. And for those M.E. sufferers who are prevented from developing any close sexual relationship at all because of the restrictions of the illness, or whose relationship has ended because of it, there is another whole area of grief, loss and loneliness to come to terms with. I feel the only way to do this, is again to try to use the experience of the illness to re-evaluate both one's own sense of self, and the range of ways in which one is able to relate to and value other people. Our society tends to emphasise the importance, above all else, of having a sexual relationship but in reality, there are lots of ways of loving other people that can be equally satisfying. If one can accept this, then one opens oneself to what is on offer, rather than using up energy in hankering after the unobtainable. Obviously this is easier said than done, and there will still be moments of acute sadness, not to mention sexual frustration, but these can at least be tempered, by masturbation on the purely physical level, and by the quality of life that can come from being completely open and responsive to all kinds of relationships with other people, and all kinds of experiences.

But what if none of this is possible? What if your M.E. is so bad that you simply cannot manage to live alone at all, never mind about such luxuries as work or relationships? What happens then?

Any solution to this will mean giving up a measure of independence, which is difficult for anyone accustomed to living alone. If your parents are fit, and able to care for you, you can then return 'home'. Alternatively, other relatives or friends may offer somewhere to live. In such situations a 'granny flat' can be a good compromise, offering carers and M.E. sufferer alike a measure of freedom, privacy and independence, whilst also affording regular care for the sufferer and mutual company/privacy for all. In such circumstances, maximum use still needs to be made of additional outside help, to ensure that neither carers nor sufferers are over-burdened, the former by practical tasks and resentments, the latter by guilt and claustrophobia.

Another solution for an M.E. sufferer unable to look after her/himself is some form of sheltered accommodation. This, however, is difficult to come by. Supply is vastly outstripped by demand. It is only those of us who have the illness very badly who are likely to qualify for a place, either in a council-run complex, a Housing Association development, or in accommodation provided by one of several voluntary organisations working in this field. It should be stressed, however, that the nature of M.E. makes it difficult for a sufferer to obtain sheltered accommodation in all but the very worst cases. Most of us do get better, even if the illness lasts a long time; most of us do have good periods in among the relapses. In this hard-pressed world of cut-backs, such fluctuations in our illness put M.E. sufferers at the end of a very long queue when it comes to obtaining sheltered housing. However, if the M.E. is really bad, and a person has nowhere to go, then a fight should be made to get an adequate placement, with help from the local housing manager, GP, consultant or social worker.

As a final point, however, it should be stressed that, even with quite bad illness, by enlisting the type of help described above, it should be possible for an M.E. sufferer not just to manage on his or her own, but also to get real enjoyment out of life, minute by minute.

2. Self-Help

So long as conventional medicine seems to be of relatively little help in altering the natural course of recovery in M.E., the onus lies on sufferers themselves to try and create the optimum conditions for progress to take place. A period of slow, steady convalescence is essential – something which has gone out of fashion in modern medicine.

REST AND RELAXATION

Rest is definitely the most important factor in promoting recovery from M.E. Without rest, recovery will *not* occur, and those patients who continually struggle on, either at home or at work, to the point of regularly reaching mental or physical fatigue stand very little chance of making any form of positive progress.

Rest means not only relaxing physically, but mentally as well. Every single day needs to be carefully planned ahead to make sure that activities are spaced to allow a period of rest in between. Ideally, rest periods should be taken in quiet surroundings where there is freedom from interruption. Take the phone off the hook; let friends and neighbours know that you usually have a rest period during the afternoon, don't want to be disturbed, and probably won't answer the doorbell.

No M.E. patient should feel guilty about taking a period of bed rest in the afternoon. For many sufferers it's the only way they can manage to complete the day. You don't have to go to sleep, just have a quiet lie down for an hour or so, and listen to the radio or tape if you don't feel sleepy. Alternatively, make it the time of day you carry out the relaxation techniques described earlier (see pages 76–7).

In the very early stages of M.E. (i.e. straight after the initial viral infection) I have no hesitation in recommending a period of *total bed rest* before a very gradual return to normal activities. This may mean two or three weeks in bed and several months getting back to normal: by doing so you will, hopefully, avoid the progression of M.E. into a chronic condition lasting for years.

However, prolonged bed rest can also damage your health, and once the disease has become established, it requires careful thought. (In my own case a period of three weeks' bed rest, two years after the original illness when the diagnosis was first made failed to produce any benefits.) Besides the obvious problems of constipation, prolonged immobility from bed rest can produce rather more serious consequences. Doctors now refer to an 'immobility syndrome' which can occur after such extended periods of rest, with decreased oxygen intake to the lungs, risks of venous thrombosis in the legs (another good reason for taking some form of passive exercise) and loss of calcium, increasing the risk of osteoporosis later. If you put a perfectly healthy person to bed for a couple of weeks, he or she will feel very weak when trying to get up and about again. It's hardly surprising that an M.E. sufferer experiences much greater difficulties when trying to return to relative normality.

Complete bed rest is only to be recommended at the time of a relapse (e.g. with another unrelated infection) or if you seem to be on a downhill patch, possibly from trying to do too much physically or mentally. At the time of relapse I immediately go to bed, and try to rest as much as possible, for say forty-eight hours, or a little longer. After that I try to start a gradual recovery process – even if it only means getting out of bed to sit in my chair for half an hour. I know it's not always possible, but the longer you do stay on bed rest during a relapse, the harder it's going to be to 'get going again'.

Some M.E. sufferers may find themselves confined to bed for quite long periods. If this is so, do try and make sure that either you or your family help with some passive exercises with your arms and legs whilst in bed. This involves carrying out the normal movements you'd make when up and about. Some people find it quite comforting to do these sort of exercises while in a warm bath. If you're not sure about what you could be doing, a physiotherapist might be willing to come in and help.

There will be times when long periods are spent confined to the bedroom – especially during a relapse. It may be worth making some significant alterations to the bedroom's layout to make it into an all-purpose room, in which you can eat, work, see visitors, as well as relax and sleep. During a period of relapse, a trip up and down the stairs can be quite shattering, so make the bedroom as comfortable as possible, with the phone by the bed. Have some shelves close by to keep books and other essential items on. Try also to transfer a few kitchen essentials, so that you don't go downstairs continually to the kitchen to get a drink or prepare a snack. It may all seem very strange to friends, relatives and visitors, but it is a very practical solution to trying to make sure you get rest when necessary.

It's a good idea, if you can afford it, to invest in a comfortable firm mattress and good pillows for the bed – after all, you're probably spending more of your life there than anywhere else. It's also quite helpful to have a comfortable armchair in the bedroom, so you can get up and sit for a while, if you don't want to venture downstairs.

Try not to get bothered about seeing your visitors in the bedroom. If the room is large enough, have a couple of fold-up chairs for visitors to use. Socialising with friends and relatives can be a tiring experience when you're not well, and this works as a compromise to not seeing people at all.

Make sure you have a good bedside light. If you like watching television consider buying a portable set for the bedroom, but try not to let it become your main interest!

During more stable periods you may still need extensive rest. If you get up in the morning and feel awful, knowing that body and mind aren't going to function effectively, do try resting or even going back to bed for a bit, and possibly start again after lunch. Don't struggle on with what you intended to do – you'll only end up making mistakes, and making yourself feel worse in the process. On the other hand, if you do start the day off well, and accomplish all that you planned to do, follow this by considering very carefully how much extra you can now do. It's far better to build up your activities gradually during a good spell, than overdo it on the first few days, and end up feeling bloody awful because you tried to do too much.

No two days are going to be the same with M.E., and predicting how one is going to feel tomorrow or the following week is quite impossible. This is why forward planning of any sort of activity becomes so difficult, and arrangements frequently have to be cancelled at the last minute.

It can be very helpful to make a written list of all planned activities for the coming week – nothing too ambitious – and then tick them off as you go along. It does help self-esteem to actually plan to do something and then carry it out, and keep some record of what you've actually done, even though it may be a shadow of your previous performance.

EXERCISE

One of the most difficult aspects of coming to terms with a new lifestyle is striking the right balance between taking an adequate amount of rest on one hand, and what might be described as 'beneficial exercise' on the other. All too often, one hears about M.E. patients – and here I include myself – who, in the earliest stages of the illness, before any diagnosis has been made, have tried to get better by overdoing exercise and not taking sufficient rest.

REST	ACTIVITY
Essential for recovery but if prolonged can be harmful	Beneficial, provided you keep within your own limitations - excess will produce a relapse

First, how much exercise should you be taking and in what form? Like everything else, exercise tolerance in M.E. varies considerably from patient to patient, but each individual soon learns to recognise his or her own limitations – be it walking, gardening or any other physical activity. The cardinal rule when taking part in any sort of activity is to avoid pushing yourself to the point of fatigue, and *never* to the point of exhaustion. In practice this is probably best explained by using a diagram:

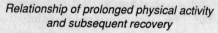

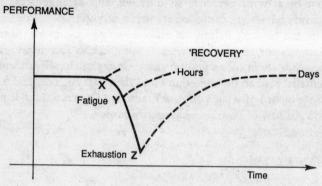

Relationship of prolonged physical activity and subsequent recovery

You know already from your own experiences that after starting to go for a walk you can carry on at a fairly steady pace till you reach **X** – when the muscles start to tire. For some sufferers this may only be 100 yards, but for others it may be half a mile or so. If you then decide to push on beyond point **X** the fatigue becomes steadily worse, till you reach a point **Y**, where it's becoming very difficult to go much further. If you still decide to carry on beyond **Y** there is a rapid deterioration, and you're very quickly exhausted and weak at the knees, forcing complete cessation of activity – **Z**.

The aim in all physical activity must therefore be to learn how much you can usefully achieve before reaching the points of fatigue and exhaustion, and keep within those limits at all times. If you stop your physical activity at or before the point of fatigue your recovery period back to normal strength should be fairly short – minutes or hours. Going to the point of exhaustion may mean that it takes days before you feel relatively normal again, and the muscle strength has returned.

WHAT SORT OF EXERCISE IS HELPFUL IN M.E.?

Few M.E. sufferers find that they can participate in any form of active sport, and certainly in nothing which involves both physical ability and rapid mental functioning. The great danger is that when going through a good patch, you may decide to go for a jog, or try a light game of tennis. Within a quarter of an hour you have to stop, exhausted, and you may now be heading for a relapse. There are, however, some physical activities which can still be carried out, as long as you're feeling reasonably well, and provided you stick to your limitations.

If you like to walk for pleasure, try to go on 'circular tours', so that you end up back at home, within your limitations. Don't set off and reach the point of fatigue half way round. You've still got to get back home again.

Some sufferers enjoy gardening, but others have had to almost abandon this pleasurable activity, because of the amount of bending and stooping involved. There are many aids that can make gardening easier, and the Society for Horticultural Therapy (see page 212) can give advice and support to people with disabilities, who find gardening very therapeutic.

Another enjoyable form of exercise is a short period of swimming in a warm pool. You may find that your local authority pool has a special weekly session when the water is heated up a little extra. The Association of Swimming Therapy promotes and teaches the art of swimming to people with disabilities using a special technique called the Halliwick Method (see page 200). The buoyancy of the water in a swimming pool makes it an ideal medium in which to exercise weakened muscles in a gentle fashion, and also to mobilise any painful joints. Your local hospital may also have a hydrotherapy pool, and a physiotherapist may be able to arrange a regular session.

Some patients also find yoga beneficial, but do take guidance from an experienced teacher, and stick to positions which are not too fatiguing.

In the end it all comes down to listening to what your body is telling you. If you're going through a good patch don't overdo it, but gradually try to increase your activities on a day-by-day basis. Don't push on at a faster pace than you can adequately cope with, or you'll just end up relapsing again.

NUTRITION

It goes without saying that all aspects of healthy eating should be encouraged in M.E., taking into account any personal allergies or sensitivities.

Many M.E. sufferers have a variety of 'digestive problems', and this may be connected with the presence of persisting enterovirus in the bowel wall, interfering with the sensitive enzymes which control digestion and absorption of food. There may be some problems with absorption of nutrients, vitamins and essential trace elements (copper, zinc, magnesium), but this hasn't yet been proved scientifically. Vitamin and mineral supplements won't do any harm provided they're not taken in excess, and could be beneficial if such deficiencies exist.

A well-balanced diet should be low in fat and sugar, and contain plenty of fresh fruit and vegetables. Some people advocate a radical change in diet, but this should only be carried out under strict medical supervision. Some M.E. patients believe that some of their problems may be due to allergies to dairy products, so they cut them out of their diet. This lack of calcium and absence of physical exercise are significant risk factors, which may make some M.E. sufferers more prone to developing osteoporosis in their later life. It's essential for anyone with M.E. – especially those who are under thirty-five – to make sure they have adequate calcium in the diet, and if necessary take some form of calcium supplement. Alternative approaches to diet, supplementation with minerals and vitamins, along with the possible role of food allergies and sensitivities are discussed in detail on pages 154–74 on alternative and complementary approaches to M.E.

HOBBIES

Non-sufferers often wonder how M.E. patients can keep themselves occupied throughout their long days stuck at home. A non-energetic hobby can be both entertaining and rewarding.

Before I got M.E. many of my interests had started to gather dust, but the stamp collection has been sorted out, and I've become interested in photography once again. Writing isn't the sort of thing that everyone can do easily, but I now know several friends with M.E. who have taken this up – it's the sort of activity you can do without much physical effort. Some people have invested in a word processor, which is also great fun, and very helpful when you can easily correct all the mistakes!

Starting a new academic course from home might be something to think about. Open University courses can be taken over a period of several years, and the organisers are keen to help people with disabilities wherever possible. (See page 209.)

Pets are a very good source of companionship. They don't chatter away all day, but can be there as a friend. Remember, a dog will need exercising. A cat (Siamese are great friends), a budgie, or even a guinea pig would do just as well.

AVOIDING A RELAPSE

Whatever the current state of your illness, be it static, recovering, or even now in remission, there's always the possibility that a relapse may occur. Most M.E. sufferers quickly learn to recognise the things which seem almost guaranteed to worsen M.E., but avoiding them isn't always easy. Undue physical and mental stress are probably the commonest causes of relapse, and these factors, along with the adverse effects of temperature extremes have already been covered. However, there are other important factors which all patients need to take care with.

ALCOHOL

Alcohol intolerance is extremely common in M.E.; I rarely see a patient who doesn't volunteer this fact, and if you're not affected by large amounts of alcohol M.E. seems an unlikely diagnosis. Some sufferers who previously enjoyed and tolerated regular consumption of alcohol, without any adverse effects, now find that even small amounts make them feel extremely unwell. This isn't an allergy but a hypersensitivity to the effects of alcohol, possibly related to two important facts.

First, the soporific effects of alcohol are partly explained by the fact that it increases the effects of one of the brain's chemicals (neurotransmitters) – gamma amino butyric acid (GABA). This in turn reduces the availability of calcium, which is responsible for triggering nerve cell activity, and so brain function is depressed.

Second, alcohol can also dilate the small blood vessels in the skin, so it helps to divert blood flow away from the brain and other vital organs. So, anyone who is particularly susceptible to the autonomic/vasomotor effects of M.E. (feeling faint or dizzy on standing up) will probably find this made worse after alcohol.

It's difficult to say whether alcohol consumption, even in moderation, causes any harm in M.E. If there's any evidence of inflammation in the liver it should be avoided altogether. However, most patients find that they no longer want any alcohol, so the problem doesn't arise.

I have come across the occasional patient who has used alcohol to try and 'blot out' their symptoms of M.E.; but this is alcohol abuse. It's a very dangerous path to start on; you only end up feeling ten times worse the next morning, and run a serious risk of becoming an alcoholic.

One final reason for avoiding alcohol is the fact that it can damage muscle, but this is usually only associated with heavy drinking.

CIGARETTES AND ENVIRONMENTAL POLLUTION

Any form of environmental pollution, and that means both active smoking and inhaling other people's smoke (passive smoking) is best avoided if at all possible. Do explain to your friends and relatives that *their* smoking might be damaging *your* health, and try to make your house or office a no-smoking zone.

Smoking cigarettes decreases the capability of the red blood cells to carry vital oxygen around the body in an efficient manner. M.E. research has already suggested that there may be problems with the red cells themselves, as well as lack of oxygen to vital muscle and nerve cells. It doesn't seem sensible to go and exacerbate this problem further.

Many M.E. patients undoubtedly feel a lot better in a non-polluted atmosphere, and it's also wise to clean up the environment at home by banning (like Prince Charles) the use of aerosols and spray-on chemicals.

DRUGS

All medication, both prescribed by your doctor, or purchased over the counter (and this includes vitamins, minerals and herbal preparations) should be taken with caution, and only with good reason. M.E. sufferers seem to experience increased sensitivity to many drugs.

DRUGS AND M.E.:

1 DRUGS WHICH MAY EXACERBATE PRE-EXISTING M.E. SYMPTOMS:

ANTIDEPRESSANTS	– worsen autonomic/vasomotor symptoms, and can cause further sedation.
TRANQUILLISERS	– increased sedating effect.
BETA-BLOCKERS	– fatigue in higher doses.
SOME ASTHMA DRUGS	– worsen autonomic symptoms.

2 DRUGS TO WHICH PATIENTS SEEM MORE SENSITIVE:
ANTIBIOTICS
SOME ANALGESICS and NSAIDs

3 DRUGS WHICH ARE BEST AVOIDED

STEROIDS	– depress the immune system.

Antibiotic sensitivity is a problem in some patients, but if you succumb to a serious infection which requires treatment with a specific antibiotic, then do take it – unless, of course, you have a true allergy to something like penicillin.

INFECTIONS

Picking up any new infection will probably increase the effects of M.E. Patients who are in regular contact with small children may find it difficult to avoid such infections. It's obviously sensible to try and avoid close contact with any friend or relative who has an infection, particularly anyone who is coughing or spluttering, even though this may seem anti-social.

Good dental care with regular check-ups is also very important, as a nasty grumbling tooth or gum infection can make you very debilitated.

If you do get any sort of infection and start to feel off-colour, rest immediately and perhaps go back to bed for forty-eight hours. It depends on how severe the infection is. Rest as necessary, and then start a recovery plan.

If you have an infection and temperature and are not sure why, it's wise to consult your general practitioner after about forty-eight hours. It may be a urinary infection or chest infection, which is producing little in the way of obvious symptoms, but may need antibiotic treatment.

A severe infection is likely to leave an M.E. sufferer feeling extra-debilitated for many weeks, so be patient while gradually returning to your usual state of health.

SURGICAL OPERATIONS AND GENERAL ANAESTHETICS

For an M.E. sufferer, having an operation will be a major event, so try to do everything possible to minimise the upheaval. To start, to be in the best physical state possible, try to get a period of forty-eight hours' solid rest before the day of admission.

Let both your consultant and anaesthetist know in advance that you have M.E.; and the effect that it has on you. Surgeons and anaesthetists probably may not know very much about M.E., so you may have to explain that it is a genuine medical problem which can be exacerbated by surgery and anaesthetics. Often, when a patient is admitted to hospital with a co-existing medical problem, and the surgical team don't know much about it, they'll ask one of their physician colleagues to come and look you over as well.

The actual surgery is probably inevitable, but there is a trend towards using less drastic methods wherever possible. Kidney stones, for example, can now be dissolved, which doesn't involve any surgery on the kidney at all, and some gall stones can be dissolved by new drugs. Such alternatives aren't available for everything, but ask your surgeon if the operation is really necessary, and whether there are any alternative approaches available.

Local anaesthesia is also being used increasingly for a whole range of operations (some of them quite major), and again this is a possibility which you can discuss with the anaesthetist.

Explain to the sister on the surgical ward that you have M.E.; and what you can and can't do for yourself. It's quite likely that they haven't nursed a patient with M.E., and like the surgeons they work with, know little about the illness. It might be worth taking in a medical article on M.E. for them to read, but the response may be very varied!

Your recovery post-operation is likely to be slower than usual. Everyone feels weak and tired after an operation, but the M.E. sufferer will probably experience increased fatigue for a much longer period. Hopefully the ward will be sympathetic, and will not try to get you going at too fast a pace. If you're not happy about things, do speak to the sister or one of the surgical doctors.

You may require a considerable degree of help when you return home, from both the family, and possibly the community nursing services. Try and make sure this sort of help is organised before you go into hospital, so that everything runs smoothly on your return home.

VACCINATIONS

Some M.E. sufferers experience a quite severe reaction or relapse in symptoms following vaccinations. The risk has to be carefully weighed up against the chances of contracting whatever disease you are protecting against. For example, maintaining up-to-date tetanus protection for a patient living on a farm would be more important than risking a reaction, and should be discussed with your doctor. On the other hand, flu vaccinations are probably better avoided, unless there is a good medical reason for having one. It's certainly important to avoid crowded public places when there is a flu epidemic in progress. The value of high doses of Vitamin C in preventing or curing colds and flu remains unproven.

Foreign travel occasionally involves compulsory vaccination, as well as those vaccinations which are just recommended. Polio is still a common disease in underdeveloped countries and it would be very unwise to go there without full protection. Typhoid and cholera vaccines offer less protection and can cause bad reactions in quite healthy people. Taking sensible precautions with food, drinking water and where you bathe is probably just as important as the vaccination. Reactions here can be reduced by having the injection just into the skin (intradermally).

Antimalarial tablets *must* be taken if advised.

For a small fee MASTA (Medical Advisory Services for Travel Abroad, Tel (01) 631 4408) operates an individual advice scheme on the prevention of illness abroad.

SUMMARY OF HOW TO COPE WITH A RELAPSE OF M.E.

- Try to avoid any of the factors which worsen M.E. already described.
- At the first sign of a relapse in your state of health, start to increase your ratio of rest to activity. If you've got an infection and temperature go to bed. Aspirin is still a very good drug to use, provided you can tolerate it.
- If you have a serious infection let your general practitioner know, and take any antibiotics prescribed.
- Organise your bedroom into a living area, so you're not struggling up and down the stairs all day.
- Try not to prolong the strict bed rest for more than a few days, and don't be afraid to commence a gradual rehabilitation programme, keeping within your limitations.

- Try to do some muscle exercises during bed rest, either by yourself or with help from family or a physiotherapist.
  Don't repeat any exercise to the point of fatigue.
  Don't exercise painful muscles and joints – let them settle down first.
- Don't neglect your diet – if you can't face solid food try to take some liquid nourishment (e.g. Complan), and don't let your fluid intake fall.
- Organise the family, friends, neighbours into helping out as much as possible.

Your body can recover from a relapse of M.E.; but you've got to give it the best possible circumstances in which to do so. And remember, it's far better to regard these relapses as setbacks on your road to recovery, rather than a 'step down the ladder'.

3. Exploring The Alternatives

ACUPUNCTURE

Acupuncture is a traditional Chinese technique which involves the insertion of very fine needles into specific points of the body – the acupuncture points.

The Chinese view of health and disease differs markedly to that of conventional western ideas. They feel that our bodies are in a state of flux between what they refer to as Yin (passivity) and Yang (activity). The healthy body is 'in balance', but the unhealthy body is 'out of balance' between these two vital forces. The aim of acupuncture is to restore balance, and so return the body to normal.

An essential part of the Chinese philosophy is that energy (Qi) flows through the body in channels, each channel corresponding to one of the vital organs such as the heart, brain, etc. If there is disease present in that part of the body then the energy flow in that specific channel is disrupted. These channels don't exist in terms of conventional anatomy. They can't be found at dissection like nerves or blood vessels, and this is why conventional medicine finds this theory hard to understand. By selecting sites where these channels of energy pass, and applying the acupuncture needle, the aim is to correct the dysfunction in energy flow.

The acupuncturist decides which parts of the body are unhealthy by first carrying out a clinical examination, not dissimilar to a normal doctor, but particular attention is paid to the pulse and the state of the tongue – considered to be key indicators of health by the Chinese.

Can acupuncture help M.E.? Conventional medicine accepts that part of the therapeutic effect of acupuncture involves the release of morphine-like substances (endorphins) in the body, which is why it can be so effective in pain relief and even anaesthesia. Perhaps it might be a good alternative for any M.E. patient who requires an anaesthetic for an operation?

Any M.E. sufferer who has particular problems with localised bone or muscle pain, unrelieved by ordinary pain killers, might well consider making use of this approach.

Another effect of acupuncture is on the autonomic nerves (which cause vasomotor instability), and again patients experiencing such symptoms (e.g. palpitations) might find acupuncture worth trying.

Acupuncture can't 'cure' something like M.E., but it could help with some symptoms. In China, acupuncture is a true form of complementary medicine, with acupuncturists working alongside colleagues in hospitals and clinics who work along traditional western lines. Acupuncture usually needs to be given in a course of treatments, if it's going to have any effect: you won't gain benefit from a one-off treatment. Benefits may not start to occur for several weeks or months, and further treatment may be necessary at a later date.

This therapy can now be obtained on the NHS, but with great difficulty. A few general practitioners have become interested and use it on their patients, but they are still few in number, and there's not much financial incentive for them to do it. A few of the NHS pain clinics also use acupuncture as part of a multidisciplinary approach. For most patients, though, it means going privately. For how to find an acupuncturist, see page 199.

ALLERGIES – ARE THEY A PART OF M.E.?

Allergies are included in this chapter on alternative approaches to M.E., as it's quite wrong to infer that M.E. is an 'allergic disease', like asthma or hay fever. Some M.E. sufferers go on to develop secondary allergies as part of the disease process (and I've suffered from hay fever since developing M.E.). However, allergies are common in a normal population of adults, with up to 15 per cent having some form of allergy, and so the association with M.E. may be just pure coincidence.

The most likely explanation for M.E. patients developing allergies seems to be the effect of persisting virus and immune disturbances unmasking allergies in an already susceptible patient. It is worrying to find that some patients, who have no evidence of allergic symptoms, are spending vast amounts of money at private allergy clinics, trying to find what they are allergic to.

Of all the alternative approaches to the management of M.E. allergies are probably the most confusing. Allergy, in medical terms, is simply a way of describing an over-enthusiastic response by the immune system to factors which most people would regard as harmless. The allergic symptoms then occur whenever a sensitive (allergic) patient comes in contact with that substance – the allergen. A comprehensive list of all known allergens would be endless, but many of them are normal everyday constituents of our environment: pollens, furs, foods, and drugs. Some truly allergic patients have allergies which change in the course of time. So, identifying which particular allergens are involved in any one individual isn't always easy.

Symptoms result from inflammatory responses taking place in different parts of the body. Inhaled allergens can cause asthma, chemicals on the skin can cause eczema, and foods can produce varied symptoms: abdominal pain, changes in bowel habit, etc. When an allergic patient comes into contact with an allergen, the immune system responds by releasing chemicals like histamine which cause an immediate inflammatory response in the particular target tissue.

Both doctors and patients experience a considerable degree of confusion and misunderstanding over the distinction between allergy and sensitivity, and this might be particularly relevant with M.E. in relation to foods. Certainly, some people have a true allergic response to certain foods, most commonly milk and dairy products, wheat and nuts, but just because a certain food makes you feel unwell doesn't mean that you're allergic to it. Caffeine, for example, in coffee will quickly upset some people due to its direct effect on the nervous system causing palpitations, tremor and a headache. But this is a direct effect of the caffeine – there's no allergic response taking place.

Many patients seem to suffer from a variety of digestive (possibly malabsorption) problems once they've developed M.E., but if there is a persisting enterovirus in the lining membrane of the bowel this could well be causing a food sensitivity right there in the gut, as opposed to an allergic reaction in the body generally.

Whatever mechanisms are involved – allergic or increased sensitivity – the most reliable way of detecting a 'culprit' food is by an exclusion diet, followed by a challenge with the suspected food, but this must be done with the help of a doctor or dietician. This type of diet involves a strict regime of what we like to call 'non-allergic foods' for a week or so. This could consist of spring water, a source of protein such as lamb, and a source of carbohydrate like rice. Foods can then be slowly introduced in groups (e.g. wheat products) to see if any one produces a recurrence of symptoms. If no significant improvement has occurred at the end of the strict exclusion, it would seem that food sensitivity or allergy is not the cause of the problem.

ALLERGY TESTING

Many patients are being led to believe that a whole range of allergies can be quickly and simply diagnosed by 'allergy tests', but this just isn't so. Conventional medicine tends to rely on the results of skin (provocation) tests and blood tests. These can be obtained on the NHS by referral to an allergy clinic at the local hospital.

Skin tests A small amount of very diluted allergen is pricked into the skin, and the inflammatory response – due to histamine release – measured. This type of testing is particularly useful for inhaled allergens causing asthma; for skin eczema; but only for a few food allergies (e.g. egg). For the majority of foods it's probably of little value as they don't tend to produce this type of response in such a short time.

Blood tests measure the levels of specific antibodies which allergic patients make in response to specific allergens. (This is known as the RAST test – standing for Radio Allego Sorbant Test.) These results again have to be carefully interpreted, as not all foods produce this type of response.

A wide variety of other allergy tests are available, but conventional allergists still regard many of them as being of dubious value, and they're not available from the NHS. Alternative investigations not yet accepted by conventional medicine include Cytotoxic tests and Neutralisation Testing.

TREATMENT OF ALLERGIES

Once an allergy or sensitivity has been found the obvious solution is to try and avoid, wherever possible, the particular allergen.

Conventional medicine treats allergies with a variety of drugs. Antihistamines, sodium cromoglycate (which covers the histamine-containing cells and prevents its release) and the powerful anti-inflammatory steroids are all used depending on the type and severity of the symptoms. Steroids are not recommended for M.E. patients unless really necessary, as they dampen down immune responses.

Non-orthodox practitioners use a variety of approaches to manage allergic disease, and again their value is heavily criticised by some doctors. A method which is used by M.E. sufferers is:

Enzyme Potentiated Transepidermal Desensitisation (EPD) This method of treating allergy was originally developed by Dr McEwan at St Mary's Hospital in London. Although only available privately, some NHS allergists are open minded about its possible value. The process involves an injection which contains a combination of an enzyme (beta glucuronidase) and a dilute mixture of numerous food allergens. The enzyme is supposed to prevent the immune system from overreacting to the food allergies in the mixture. The treatment has to be administered several times during the first year, and then boosters are given at increasing intervals depending on the individual patient's response.

The subject of allergies and M.E. creates a considerable amount of heated debate between those who support the theories and others who don't see allergies as having much to do with this illness. This is undoubtedly very confusing for patients, who can't follow the scientific arguments, and are baffled by what they ought to do. I've tried to present the facts as I see them. I don't accept that allergic reactions are a major part of M.E.; although there are some patients who have allergies (or sensitivities), and identification and correct management could help them feel a lot better.

AROMATHERAPY

Here, small quantities of various plant oils are used, although these can be quite expensive. This therapy is undoubtedly very soothing and relaxing, especially using an oil such as Lavender in the bath, but I feel it is unlikely to produce anything more than symptomatic relief.

CANDIDA ALBICANS

Candida is a yeast-like fungus, commonly present in various parts of the body, in perfectly healthy people. Then, for the reasons already described on pages 59–61 (vaginal thrush in secondary problems) it gets out of control and starts to cause various symptoms. Besides vaginal thrush it can also occur:

- In the mouth there may be little white patches on the lining membrane. In very debilitated people this infection can also spread down to the oesophagus, and cause serious problems.
- Skin infections, particularly affecting areas which are warm and moist, which is the sort of environment candida thrives in. Hands and nails which are constantly in water are very prone to infection, but it can also affect skin elsewhere on the body.
- In truly debilitated patients, such as someone with a severe immunedeficiency like AIDS, the candida overgrowth can cause problems in the lungs.

159

However, at this point conventional and alternative medical opinion often part company. The latter believes that candida overgrowth can then go on to play a part in a whole range of chronic illnesses such as multiple sclerosis, rheumatoid arthritis and M.E. They also believe that candida in the gut can be responsible for a diverse spectrum of digestive symptoms ranging from excess wind and bloating to abdominal pain. They further believe that candida causes the gut lining to leak and produces harmful toxins which can affect the immune system. These toxins pass to the brain (where they are said to produce some of the brain malfunction seen in M.E.) and even some of the hormone producing glands in the body.

It must be said that the majority of conventional microbiologists are not at all convinced by these claims, and they spend much of their working lives studying such organisms. When I've sought the views of other doctors involved in M.E. research on this aspect of management, many of them express opinions which range from open-minded scepticism to outright hostility. Patients who therefore decide to try out such an anti-candida regime will have to accept that their general practitioners are likely to adopt similar attitudes, and may even refuse to co-operate in prescribing the anti-candida medication, which you can't buy from the pharmacy without prescription. These requests may also reinforce their mistaken view that M.E. isn't a real disease.

Orthodox medical opinion argues that it's possible to find the presence of candida in almost anyone, provided you look hard enough. But simply demonstrating that candida is there is not the same as showing that it's causing a significant problem. It's only when there's evidence of overgrowth that most doctors would accept that M.E. patients are having the sort of serious problems already referred to. Rightly or wrongly, these are the attitudes of conventional doctors which will be put to you if you claim that you need to get rid of candida before you can get rid of M.E.

TREATMENT

Those who believe that it's essential to remove candida as part of an M.E. treatment regime rely on an approach which involves diet, conventional anti-fungal medication and other additional supplements.

DIET

The theory is that to help eradicate candida your diet will have to be free from both sugar and yeast, which denies the organism its essential nutrients. This sort of diet will involve cutting out foods like bread (which contains yeast), sugar and honey. Even your B vitamins have to be yeast free. Some practitioners also advocate a low carbohydrate diet to accompany this, but don't start this sort of dietary manipulation by yourself without proper supervision.

DRUGS

Anti-fungal medication, such as nystatin, needs to be prescribed by your general practitioner. Nystatin is the generic name, so it comes in a variety of preparations using different trade names – e.g. Nystan. It can be used as a cream or pessary for vaginal infections, drops and pastilles for thrush in the mouth, skin creams, tablets for bowel infections as well as powder. The powder form is taken between meals, and the dose is gradually altered according to the individual response.

Nystatin appears to be a perfectly safe drug, but like any medicine it should be used with caution during pregnancy.

One anti-fungal preparation, which M.E. patients use occasionally is ketoconazole (Nizoral). This drug is potentially *very toxic* to the liver, and I don't believe it should be used by anyone with M.E., unless there are very strong medical indications to do so.

A variety of other anti-fungal preparations are also used by the practitioners who carry out this form of therapy, some of them originating abroad.

ADDITIONAL SUPPLEMENTS

Lactobacillus acidophilus is a natural constituent of the bowel, and its presence helps to keep candida in check. It can be killed off by taking antibiotics, but restored by eating 'live' yogurt (from health food shops), or can be taken in tablet form.

Other additional supplements sometimes recommended include high doses of Vitamin C, as well as other vitamins and minerals. High-dose Vitamin C will produce diarrhoea, and it's claimed this will aid the removal of candida. This megadose therapy isn't without side-effects (see vitamins, pages 164–7) and shouldn't be stopped abruptly.

Anti-fungal candida treatment isn't a scientifically proven method of managing M.E. The exponents of this therapy don't claim it will cure M.E., but that it will help to make some people feel substantially better. Certainly, there are reports of patients apparently benefiting from this approach, although others say they feel worse. Some conventional doctors are looking at the relation between yeasts and specific bowel diseases, but this research is still in its early stages and it is too soon to draw any conclusions from it.

Further information on this approach can be found in previous copies of the M.E. Association Newsletters.

DIETARY SUPPLEMENTATION

Some practitioners advocate that M.E. patients should be encouraged to supplement their diets with a variety of trace elements, amino acids and vitamins. This type of approach is particularly popular in America for a variety of illnesses; once again the theories are quite attractive, although there is little evidence to back them up and win the acceptance of orthodox medicine.

The idea behind this approach is that there may be both faulty absorption of some of these essential substances, as well as an extra requirement to help in the repair process of essential cells which have been damaged by the persisting virus or immune malfunction. A comprehensive list of all these substances would be endless, as differing practitioners recommend their own individual treatment regimes, often using a combination of therapies. However, two trace elements, magnesium and zinc, which are quite frequently taken by M.E. sufferers, do warrant some appraisal.

Patients who are interested in this type of approach, and want to follow it up can have tests done on various mineral levels in the body by: BIOLAB, The Stone House, 9 Weymouth Street, London W1N 3FF. Tel (01) 636 5959. They are a private pathology laboratory who specialise in this type of work.

Magnesium There's no evidence that patients with M.E. are deficient in magnesium, or that taking extra amounts will affect the illness, but some practitioners do recommend its use. Magnesium deficiency has been implicated in a wide selection of illnesses including high blood pressure and pre-menstrual syndrome. However, researchers are still uncertain as to the exact roles of magnesium in the body. It certainly seems to be involved inside muscle and nerve cells helping energy metabolism, as well as being an important constituent of many enzymes.

Normal dietary intake is probably related to a person's total calorie intake as opposed to any one specific source. However, foods which are particularly rich in magnesium include green vegetables, chocolate and cereal grains. Blood tests for magnesium measure its concentration in the red blood cells.

Zinc is another trace element which is essential for the correct functioning of many of the body's enzyme systems.

Orthodox medicine acknowledges that severe deficiency can occur (often as a result of poor absorption due to conditions like cystic fibrosis), and this can cause inflamed skin lesions, increased susceptibility to infection and general failure to thrive in children.

Most people eating a normal balanced diet, containing meat and dairy produce, have a zinc intake well within the World Health Organization's recommendations. Fruit and vegetables are low in zinc, but vegetarians don't seem to be deficient.

The level of zinc in the blood is not thought to be an accurate indicator of zinc levels overall, as only a small amount is actually in the blood. Any chronic infection will probably reduce the level of zinc in the blood, but it seems that the total amount of zinc in the body doesn't fall significantly, so concluding that someone with M.E. has a mild zinc deficiency from a blood test isn't necessarily a logical conclusion.

Experimentally, zinc can interfere with virus multiplication. Even so, there's no evidence that it stops the progression of the common cold (for which it's often recommended) or any other persisting viral infection. Some allergists believe that patients with food allergy or sensitivity have an abnormal ratio of copper to zinc status in the body, and that if this is corrected there can be a considerable improvement in food-related symptoms.

Taking extra zinc isn't without side-effects (stomach pains and decreased copper absorption) and very high intakes can actually start to impair the immune system.

At present, many of the claims made for zinc supplementation are unfounded, but taking a little extra probably does no harm. No M.E. patient should take any more than 50 mgm per day (Zincomed capsules contain this dose) if they decide to use this as part of their treatment. Zinc supplements should *not* be taken by any patient who has kidney problems.

VITAMINS

Vitamins taken in normal recommended doses are extremely safe. There isn't any good evidence to say that M.E. patients are lacking in any specific vitamins, provided they're taking an adequate diet. I'm not convinced that taking extra vitamins will aid recovery, but on the other hand it won't do any harm, so it may be worth trying.

It is worrying to see the current trend towards taking vastly excessive doses of vitamins for a variety of chronic illnesses, including M.E. Some of these compounds are far from being harmless when taken in such high doses; we're not sure about the long-term effects of doing this, and unfortunately information to this effect is often lacking on the labelling or in the books and articles which recommend this approach.

This megavitamin theory is an offshoot of 'Orthomolecular

psychiatry', which is attributed to the famous scientist, Linus Pauling – the great advocate for Vitamin C. Pauling argued that many psychiatric illnesses were the result of specific biochemical abnormalities, which could be corrected by massive dietary supplementation. There is a good scientific basis to this idea, and researchers are looking for specific deficiencies in conditions like schizophrenia, but this theory has now been extrapolated to cover an ever increasing range of illness.

There are occasions when megavitamin therapy is necessary: for example, some alcoholics become severely deficient in B vitamins and get neurological problems as a result, but self-medication using this approach can lead to toxic reactions and isn't to be recommended.

VITAMINS: RECOMMENDED DAILY REQUIREMENTS FOR ADULTS

VITAMIN A 700 iu

VITAMIN B GROUP: *THIAMINE* (B1) 1.4 mgm
           RIBOFLAVIN (B2) 2.1 mgm
           NICOTINAMIDE (B3) 14 mgm
           PYRIDOXINE (B6) 2.1 mgm
           CYANOCOBALAMIN (B12) 2.0 micrograms
           BIOTIN 350 micrograms
           PANTOTHENIC ACID 14 mgm

VITAMIN C (ascorbic acid) 35 mgm, but higher in disease

VITAMIN D (calciferol) 100 iu

VITAMIN E 30 iu

FOLIC ACID 2 mgm

Vitamin toxicity It used to be thought that the water-soluble vitamins (the B and C group) could be taken in large doses without any possible harm, as the body would just flush any unrequired out in the urine. Unfortunately it's now recognised that this simple way of removing any excess isn't quite right, and harm can come from taking too much Vitamin B6 and from Vitamin C. However, it's the fat-soluble vitamins (A, D, E, K) which can accumulate and cause really serious problems, particularly Vitamin A.

Vitamin A toxicity can occur at doses not much higher than the recommended daily dose, and the effects include raised pressure in the brain and liver damage.

Vitamin B3 needs to be used with care as well, as it can cause liver damage.

Vitamin B6 is commonly used for pre-menstrual tension and many M.E. patients take it as a supplement. It's perfectly safe at low doses, but this should be kept below 150 mgm per day, as above this level toxic effects including neuritis and lack of co-ordination can occur.

Vitamin B12 is taken by some patients in injection form. It's a very effective treatment for neurological problems where there's a proven deficiency as in pernicious anaemia. There's no evidence that M.E. patients have problems with Vitamin B12 absorption or have low levels of B12 in the body, but some patients do seem to derive benefit, and it can't do any harm.

Vitamin C There is some evidence that people with a variety of chronic illnesses may have increased requirements of Vitamin C, and so there's no harm in taking a little extra, e.g. 100 mgm a day. Large doses of Vitamin C have recently become popular in America (where they are administered by injection) and over here it's sometimes used as part of an anti-candida treatment.

Although adequate intake of Vitamin C is vital for the correct functioning of the immune system, there's no scientific evidence that extra amounts can give it a boost and overcome existing problems. Experiments using animals show that Vitamin C can alter immune function, but it's not clear that these sort of effects have any relevance to humans and conditions like M.E.

One of the possible problems of continually taking very high doses of Vitamin C (i.e. more than 5 grams per day) is that this will increase the output of certain chemicals in the urine (uric acid and oxalates) which can then cause kidney stones in sus-ceptible patients, as well as giving false positive tests for sugar in the urine, causing a doctor to query diabetes. Second, as the body becomes conditioned to these very high levels of Vitamin

C it speeds up its removal mechanism in order to cope, and then if the patient suddenly stops taking it, increased removal continues and leads to a rebound scurvy. So, it's very important never to abruptly cease taking high-dose Vitamin C – always ease off gradually.

Vitamin D excess will increase levels of body calcium which can cause kidney stones and muscle weakness. The importance of maintaining an adequate level of dietary calcium was discussed on page 59.

Vitamin E levels about 600 iu per day are reported to increase blood fats and decrease levels of thyroid hormones, as well as causing stomach upsets. Above 800 iu muscle weakness can occur along with headaches and dizziness.

A multitude of claims have been made for Vitamin E, and that many M.E. sufferers take it regularly. I used to do so myself, but began to wonder if its benefits outweighed its possible side-effects, and decided to stop.

So, vitamin therapy is very popular and many claims are made. These substances need to be taken with the same caution as any medicine if you're going to go above the normal daily recommended doses. They can cause harm in megadoses, so do be careful and take proper advice. It could well be that the body doesn't need any of this sort of supplementation, and all that we're doing is making the drug companies even richer and producing some of the most expensive urine in the world, as our bodies naturally remove what we don't need!

HEALING

The term healing covers a wide variety of different therapies, the theory being that patients can be healed by 'forces' which the healer possesses, and which can be passed on to the patient. Many of these healers make strong religious claims in connection with their work, assuming, rightly or wrongly, that their powers are 'God given'. In practice the process of healing usually involves the laying on of hands, or some form of physical contact, although some healers claim to be able to transmit these healing powers by way of thought.

There seems to be an ever growing number of healers. Some of them are obviously frauds, so if you do decide to embark on healing do make careful enquiries first and try to find a genuine and respected healer. This 'mind over matter' approach can be of great value to some people, and obviously the chances of success are greatly increased if you believe in the healer and the principles of healing.

Patients who have strong religious beliefs (and even those who don't) may gain considerable benefit and comfort from Christian healing. Some churches now have specific 'healing services' as part of their worship, and your vicar will know of any which occur locally. Part of the service usually involves the priest giving an individual blessing along with the laying on of hands for those who require healing. Relatives are also very welcome to attend and to pray for recovery.

Some healers belong to the National Federation of Spiritual Healing (see page 205), but the best way of finding a healer would be by personal recommendation.

HERBAL MEDICINES

A recent survey in the *British Medical Journal* found that general practitioners understood less about herbal medicines than any other branch of alternative medicine. This is disquieting, because many of the drugs used by orthodox medicine are derived from plants, and some of the herbal medicines available for purchase have some disturbing side-effects if not used with care.

Herbalists are generally unqualified, although a few have taken some formal training. They will recommend and prepare herbal medicines for patients, but most people seem to use this branch of alternative medicine on a 'do-it-yourself' basis, by purchasing the remedies from health food stores – often without knowing a great deal about the product they're about to use. There is a vast range of herbal medicines available, and the current position with regard to licensing and control seems far from satisfactory. Patients are taking substances of which the long-term effects, in some cases, have never been properly assessed.

Although the majority are probably quite safe, some herbs are known to accumulate heavy metals and pesticide residues – which can be passed on to the patient. A few are known to cause cancer in animals (Comfrey and Sassafras) or produce severe liver damage in humans (Ragwort or 'bush tea'). Ginseng, which is quite popular among a few M.E. patients, is reported to cause high blood pressure, breast development in men (it can affect hormone levels) and 'nervous irritability'. Its proven benefits are far from certain.

There is no dispute that many of these herbs do have genuine and beneficial pharmacological effects, which is why Evening Primrose oil (Efamol) merits some serious consideration.

Evening Primrose oil has become an increasingly popular treatment for a whole range of conditions, ranging from pre-menstrual tension to rheumatoid arthritis, atopic eczema and multiple sclerosis.

Evening Primrose oil comes from seeds of the shrub *Oenothera biennis*. It's usually combined with Vitamin E, which helps to preserve the effectiveness of the oil once inside the cells. The oil is rich in two essential fatty acids. These are known as essential because our bodies can't manufacture them, and we have to take them in the diet. It's thought that these fatty acids play a part in chemical pathways that eventually have an effect on the body's immune system and inflammation responses.

There's no doubt that Evening Primrose oil has a number of firm supporters in orthodox medicine, and trials have recently been carried out to compare its effectiveness in relieving the pain in arthritis with traditional pain killers. The results seem to show it can be just as effective. There's also some good evidence that it can help quite a lot in skin conditions like eczema. In patients who are experiencing joint pain this drug might well be worth trying, especially as it doesn't have any nasty side-effects.

Many M.E. patients take Evening Primrose oil, although there is no evidence that it can alter the natural course of M.E. Until we understand much more about the immune response in

M.E. it's difficult to be sure what role such substances play, and whether Evening Primrose oil may be a worthwhile part of the treatment.

The oil usually comes in capsule form (250 mgm or 500 mgm). It is available from pharmacies and health food stores under a variety of trade names, and is quite expensive. It has recently been made available on NHS prescription, but only for the treatment of eczema.

HOMEOPATHY

Homeopathy was developed by Dr Samuel Hahnemann nearly 200 years ago. It's based on the principle that 'like cures like', and involves the use of very dilute preparations, which in a healthy person would cause specific symptoms, but could cure the same symptoms in someone who was ill. For example, because scarlet fever resembles belladonna poisoning, a very dilute dose of belladonna would be used to treat scarlet fever.

Homeopathic medicines are usually made from natural sources such as plants, minerals or animal products. The remedy is made by a process called potentisation, so that as the original solution (the 'Mother Tincture') is made more dilute, its effect is increased. Conventional medical thinking finds it difficult to understand how such a product could then be beneficial in purely scientific terms, as there's almost nothing left in the final preparation, now so diluted.

Homeopaths tend to take an holistic approach to patients and their illnesses, and will adjust the treatment to each individual case. There's no one homeopathic remedy for something like M.E. Homeopathic treatment depends on you and your individual symptoms. It's not a do-it-yourself type of alternative therapy.

Homeopathic preparations appear to be perfectly safe and free from side-effects. Many M.E. patients make use of them and some patients claim to benefit.

HYPNOSIS

Hypnosis can't and won't 'cure' M.E., but for patients who are experiencing considerable degrees of anxiety and apprehension about particular symptoms, or the condition in general, it may be of help for relaxation, and in coming to terms with M.E., instead of fighting against it. So, it may be appropriate and helpful with some of the emotional difficulties encountered with M.E., or occasionally with a specific symptom such as chronic pain.

Do remember, though, that hypnosis in the wrong hands can do a great deal of harm, especially if it's inappropriately used for psychiatric problems like severe depression. This is one form of alternative therapy which can do harm, and if you're considering using this approach I'd strongly suggest discussing it with your own doctor first. Any M.E. patient should consult a medically qualified hypnotherapist, and certainly not one out of the Yellow Pages. An increasing number of general practitioners are using hypnotherapy in their practices. One of the partners in your own practice may be interested. (See also page 207.)

MEDITATION

Some M.E. patients gain benefit from the way meditation can relax the body and mind. Meditation can take any form you like, from the type of relaxation techniques described on pages 76–7 to Christian meditation, transcendental meditation or Zen meditation. Meditation seems particularly appropriate for patients whose stressful life continually exerts a powerful negative effect on their body's ability to recover.

Probably the best-known meditation technique is transcendental meditation (TM), which was originally brought to wide public attention by the Maharishi Mahesh in the 1960s. TM is based on principles commonly used in India, and which probably date back to well before the time of Buddha, over 2,500 years ago. It involves spending periods of about twenty minutes, twice each day, sitting in a perfectly relaxed state in a quiet room, with eyes closed and breathing easily. The aim is to use the mind to settle and slow down the body, creating 'inner stillness', using a special repetitive technique called a mantra. This can be a sound, or a repeated word or phrase, which is specially chosen to suit that individual. Once started TM needs to be continued on a regular daily basis, as the effect is cumulative – it's not a one-off form of therapy.

There's no doubt that this form of 'mind over matter' can reduce the heart rate and blood pressure, and it's possible that these purely physical effects may in turn be producing beneficial psychological ones as well.

TM is quite an easy technique to acquire after you've been instructed by a trained teacher. This will usually involve going through a series of introductory talks, followed by individual sessions on the actual learning process. After that you can continue on your own.

NATUROPATHY

This therapy aims to use the body's natural internal healing powers as a basis for recovery from ill health, and makes little use of external treatments. Naturopaths tend to regard their role as helping the patient to heal themselves – so they tend to pay much more attention to the individual than the disease.

Dietary modification, with the use of fresh and unprocessed food, is one of the most important recommendations in change of lifestyle, but herbal medicines, manipulation and massage may also be included.

Part of the process of coming to terms with, and recovering from M.E., involves making changes in lifestyle, and if a naturopath fully understands the condition, they may be able to offer some helpful advice. For how to find a naturopath, see page 209.

OSTEOPATHY AND CHIROPRACTIC

Probably the commonest reason for patients consulting osteopaths is back pain, which is often related to problems with the bony vertebrae themselves or the structures which surround and support them – the muscles and ligaments.

The osteopath becomes skilled in detecting positional changes in the vertebrae, and the way that they move in relation to one another. Like the chiropractor he aims to correct these abnormalities, and hence the symptoms which occur as a result, although the practical approach of the osteopath is somewhat gentler. Both osteopaths and chiropractors first carry out a careful clinical examination, and may also make use of X-rays to exclude any conditions which could be worsened by manipulative techniques.

Many M.E. patients have back pains along with muscle spasm and pain, and if this seems to be unrelieved by conventional medical approaches these are therapies which might be worth considering. If you do have any sort of back pain it's very advisable to discuss the use of manipulative therapy with your general practitioner before going ahead. Back pain in an elderly patient with M.E. could be due to osteoporosis, in which case manipulation wouldn't be a good idea. Many general practitioners now accept osteopathy as a valid form of treatment – in fact many of them use it themselves for their bad backs, and a few have even become qualified osteopaths. Osteopathy, however, is not available on the NHS.

Qualified osteopaths have to complete a comprehensive training, and then conform to professional standards. Unfortunately, as in other forms of alternative treatment there are unqualified people calling themselves osteopaths, who may end up doing more harm than good. For how to find an osteopath, see page 209.

Chiropractors use a variety of manipulative techniques based on the assumption that the cause of symptoms such as back pain or referred nerve pain (e.g. sciatica down the leg) results from what they term 'misalignments' or subluxations of the spinal column. They believe that by correcting these misalignments they can then restore the normal anatomy, and so relieve the symptoms, be they due to muscle spasm, bone misplacement or pressure on the nerves as they pass out of the spaces between the vertebrae.

Unfortunately anybody can set up in practice and call themselves a chiropractor, and just like osteopathy in the wrong hands this can have its dangers. Registered and trained chiropractors belong to a professional organisation, and there are a few medically qualified ones. For how to find a chiropractor, see page 202.

PART 4: APPENDICES

1. Additional Help And Benefits Available in Britain

REGISTERING AS DISABLED

One of the first things you can consider doing to get additional help, is to register yourself as disabled, with your local authority. This is not the same as being registered as disabled for employment purposes – you can, in fact, do both if you wish to. After contacting the social services department, this will then involve an appointment with either a social worker or occupational therapist to assess your disability. They can come and do this at your own home if you wish.

Registering is quite voluntary, but it can help you obtain certain benefits which the local authority administers (concessionary bus fares or an orange parking badge, etc.). It also gives your local authority some idea of the number of disabled people in their locality, what their needs are, and to what extent they're meeting those needs. The actual benefits aren't great, but the more people who do register, the more pressure 'the disabled' as a group can put on both central and local government to take notice of their problems. So, by registering, you're not only helping yourself.

Financial benefits may also include help with rates and some social security benefits.

Local authorities can help with advice (and sometimes finance) on adaptations to the home, and in certain circumstances provide rate relief for disabled people. 'Rate Relief for Disabled Persons' is a leaflet which should be available from the rates department of your local council.

Financial help for alterations is very limited, but anyone who is a tenant in council property should qualify if they have a good case, for say, a wheelchair ramp.

Social workers should know about all the services that a local authority can and should provide; if you're not happy with the response from the council's officials phone the local social services department and ask to speak to the relevant social worker.

You can also approach your local councillor or citizens advice bureau if you're not satisfied by their response.

Local authorities also administer home helps, Meals on Wheels, transport concessions, and orange parking badges.

Home helps are very sought after, and often not available! The home help organiser at your local social services office will be able to give you further information. If you are able to obtain this help you'll probably have to pay part of the cost, unless you're on a very low income. Due to demand often exceeding supply you'll probably only qualify for local authority help if you're living alone (or with a relative who isn't very fit) and quite constantly disabled by your M.E., so unable to do most household tasks. Here a doctor's letter will be of help. What they actually do in the home should be suited to your particular needs, but it can include helping with cooking, cleaning and shopping.

If you can't get help from the local authority you can always try to find someone by advertising in the local shop or newspaper, or ask around to see if a neighbour has a home help who might be prepared to work a few extra hours each week.

Meals on Wheels This service operates in most parts of the country, but again tends to be overstretched, so has to be limited to those in real need, who aren't well enough to be up and about to shop and cook a hot meal every day. The service operates on weekdays only, and a small charge is made. The quality of the food is usually very good. Contact your local social services for further information.

One alternative is to make use of restaurants who are providing home delivery of pizzas, etc. It is costly, but it does mean you can have a hot meal if you can't face cooking yourself. If you've got a freezer, and are living alone, check out the already prepared meals for one, which can be kept in store.

Social workers offer a wide variety of practical help and advice. They don't just spend their time dealing with problems. They may be able to put you in touch with an appropriate agency or help you steer the correct path through the minefield of DHSS benefits.

Many social workers are experienced in listening to people who have a multitude of difficulties – financial, social, emotional, medical, etc. – and don't see any way out of their predicament. If you feel you've got to this stage, it's often very useful to sit down and talk about your anxieties with someone like a social worker, who's detached from the situation, yet has helped many others in similar circumstances. They should know all about the local authority services which are available, and may possibly 'negotiate' with the relevant department on your behalf. They also tend to have good contacts with local community and volunteer groups.

Some social workers are now attached on a part-time basis to general practitioner health centres, but the best way to contact one is to phone the local social services department and ask for an appointment, or a home visit if necessary.

District Nurses are nurses (sometimes with non-qualified helpers) who have undertaken extra training to become expert in the problems of nursing patients at home. For an M.E. patient who is spending long periods in bed they can offer practical advice to the carer on how to lift correctly, as well as assisting with bathing and dressing if there's nobody else to help someone living alone. They can also advise on what other sources of help may be locally available, and provide aids such as sheepskin mattresses to help prevent bed sores, hoists for the bathroom, bath seats, etc. The best way to make contact is via your general practitioner.

Physiotherapists don't just work in hospitals; they also work with patients out in the community. Active physiotherapy isn't usually part of M.E. rehabilitation and can even be harmful, but a physiotherapist who knows about M.E. and what isn't good for M.E. patients could be of great help. If you're on prolonged bed rest a physiotherapist could come in and show you how to carry out passive exercises on the arm and limb muscles, to stop them becoming too weak. Physiotherapists can also help with advice on wheelchairs, and what sort of walking aids may be available, e.g. Zimmer frames.

Ask your general practitioner if there is a community physiotherapist available.

Occupational Therapists work in both hospital and out in the community, where they're employed by the local authority. You can contact your local occupational therapist directly (without a doctor's letter) at the local social services department. They will then probably come and visit you at home to assess and advise you on ways in which your daily living can be made easier. Occupational therapists are quite used to advising clients about aids to help with washing, bathing, dressing, etc., as well as equipment for the kitchen and the possibility of making more major alterations to the home.

If you're going to start making life easier in the way your home is run, you'll have to accept that a whole range of domestic duties aren't going to be carried out as often, or perhaps as efficiently, as they used to be. If you find standing and carrying out tasks particularly difficult, try to sit down whenever possible. It's obviously not so easy to do the cooking, washing-up or ironing from a seated position, but it may be the only practical way to complete the task. Here, an occupational therapist can help with advice on lowering of work surfaces and suitable high seating.

Opticians can also do home visits. Your local family practitioner committee will know if this is possible.

Prescription charges M.E. patients don't qualify for exemption from these charges because of the illness, but you may do so if you're on a low income or claiming income support. For more information get a leaflet from the post office. Alternatively, if you have to get several prescriptions each month, on a regular basis, consider paying for a 'season ticket' – unlimited prescriptions for a set charge.

Public Services British Gas, British Telecom and the Electricity Boards have all become much more aware of the needs of disabled customers, and may be able to help with special adaptations to their equipment (e.g. easier knobs on a gas cooker) or, in the case of British Gas, offer free safety checks if you are registered as disabled.

FURTHER SOURCES OF PRACTICAL HELP

The Disabled Living Foundation This is probably the most important, and now has over twenty disabled living centres throughout the country. (Full list on page 204.)

The Foundation now has well over 10,000 different technical aids for the disabled on its database, and many of these can be seen on display at the living centres. At these centres patients, carers and health care professionals can find out what's available, and where they can buy or hire such equipment. The centres don't actually sell anything on display. Occupational therapists and physiotherapists are on hand to give advice on aids for any individual problem. This can be for any aspect of daily living, indoors or outdoors, ranging from those designed to help with bathing and dressing, to highly sophisticated electronic aids for the severely disabled. There's no charge made to visit the centre, and they're usually open weekdays from 9.30 to 5.30.

You don't require a doctor's referral, although the staff do like you to phone or write beforehand to arrange a fixed appointment, so they can give individual attention. If you've got a severe disability associated with M.E. it's useful to have a doctor's letter as well, giving some information on your medical state.

Disabled Information and Advice Line (DIAL) Provides locally based information on how to obtain aids. There are numerous local centres, listed in the phone book. (See page 203.)

Royal Association for Disability and Rehabilitation (RADAR) can offer advice on a whole range of issues affecting the disabled, and they publish a number of useful books. (See page 210.)

British Red Cross Local branches (see phone book) can make short-term loans of aids such as wheelchairs and commodes. They publish a helpful booklet, *Home-made Aids for Handicapped People*, price 50p.

Centre on the Environment for the Handicapped will give free advice if you are considering extending or making some major alterations to the home. They are in contact with the sort of architects who are interested and experienced in this type of work. (See page 201.)

The DHSS publish a leaflet 'Equipment for the Disabled' (Code HB2), which is available from DHSS supplies. (See page 202.)

Equipment for the Disabled publish a series of illustrated booklets on a wide range of disability problems, and act as a reference source for aids and equipment. (See page 204.)

Volunteer Bureaux exist in many areas and aim to put anyone with disabilities in touch with willing, able-bodied helpers, who are prepared to help with a very wide variety of tasks. Your Citizens Advice Bureau will know if there are local groups operating, and they sometimes have a list of volunteers available and jobs to be done printed in the local weekly paper. If you've got a specific task which needs doing, e.g. some gardening, decorating, or help with getting to the shops each week, get in touch with your local bureau organiser. They may have someone willing to help.

Care Attendant Schemes are being increasingly organised by both local authorities and voluntary organisations. They will provide paid helpers who try to help disabled people with a wide range of tasks on a fairly flexible basis. The type of care provided can be on a personal basis, e.g. helping with washing or dressing, or more general tasks in the home. Such help is probably only available for M.E. sufferers who are quite badly affected, and either living alone or being looked after by a carer who also isn't in the best of health. This sort of service doesn't occur everywhere, but your local social services department or Citizens Advice Bureau will know if it does.

THE DHSS: SICKNESS AND OTHER BENEFITS AVAILABLE

You may find that you need to make use of state social security benefits which are available if you're out of work. You contribute taxes throughout your lifetime, so now there shouldn't be any feeling of guilt in claiming benefits if necessary. Unfortunately, even though M.E. is a genuine illness, some examining medical officers still aren't up to date with the facts on M.E., and don't always see it that way.

On the positive side, there's no doubt that there has been a significant change in the way the DHSS views M.E. as an illness, and the disability it causes. Claims for benefit are being considered in a more sympathetic manner, and sufferers don't any longer have to get their doctors to write some form of psychiatric diagnosis on the sick note in order to get the benefit. And, in a recent House of Commons reply (*Hansard*, 27 November 1987) Mrs Edwina Currie MP stated, quite clearly, that 'the National Health Service recognises and treats the disease' (M.E.).

The different benefits, and rules governing your eligibility, are often complex, and sometimes misunderstood by the people who administer them. If you are in any doubt about your eligibility, do make a written claim and see what happens – it can't do any harm, providing you're not being dishonest in the information you provide. If your application is refused, don't give up, and make an appeal if this is possible – after all, you're not only fighting for yourself, but for other M.E. sufferers in the same position as well.

If it becomes necessary to appeal against a DHSS decision, some lawyers aren't very well informed or helpful, and it's often better to 'do it yourself' with the help of a disabled rights organisation or trade union.

Some of the best impartial advice can be obtained from the various disability rights organisations such as the Disability Alliance, local Citizens Advice Bureaux and Welfare Rights Centres set up by local authorities. There are some very useful handbooks published by these organisations – see page 218.

Some practical advice on dealing with the DHSS (and other parts of officialdom)

- Always try to find out who you are talking to, either on the phone, or at an interview.
- Preferably do things by letter, and always keep your own, dated copy of any correspondence. If you're sending important documents keep a photocopy of them in case they get lost, and post them by recorded delivery. If you deal with the office by phone, always make a note in your diary about what was said, and by whom.
- If you want to discuss something at the office, phone to make an appointment, and if you're not happy about tackling officials by yourself, take a friend or relative along as well. There shouldn't be any objection if you explain your disability.
- Make a written note of what you want to ask before you go, and then record the official's replies.

- If you're not happy with the answers, ask to speak to a supervisor of the relevant department, or write a letter to the manager.
- If you're getting nowhere with a claim, a letter to your MP (at the House of Commons, London SW1) will be passed on to the local DHSS office with a request for a swift reply. As a last resort I've written to the Minister himself (at the DHSS, Whitehall, London SW1), and if this doesn't work a letter to Her Majesty the Queen can be extremely effective in making officialdom move!

GUIDE TO INDIVIDUAL BENEFITS

DHSS benefits for the sick and disabled fall into three broad categories:

1 Those which help replace income for anyone who is no longer able to work:
  Statutory Sick Pay
  Invalidity Benefit
  Severe Disablement Allowance – if you've no national insurance contributions.
2 Benefits providing extra help for the severely disabled are:
  Attendance Allowance
  Invalid Care Allowance
  Home Responsibilities Protection
3 Benefit to help increase mobility:
  Mobility Allowance.
(See also section on increasing mobility, pages 102–9.)

STATUTORY SICK PAY

At the onset of any illness, providing you're at work, you'll receive Statutory Sick Pay (SSP) from your employer, which may then be 'topped up' to a percentage of normal pay, depending on how long you've been employed.

INVALIDITY BENEFIT

For people who have been incapable of work for the past twenty-eight weeks, and previously claiming Statutory Sick Pay (SSP) from their employer, or a non-contributory sickness benefit. It's still possible to claim Invalidity Benefit, if you haven't been claiming SSP. This may apply to some self-employed, and unemployed as well as widows/widowers. Payment can continue till 65 (women) and 70 (men).

The total, non-taxable, weekly payment is made up of three separate parts:

a) Invalidity Pension which gives a payment for the claimant, plus allowances for dependants. If a wife or husband earns (after expenses) more than a certain amount per week, his or her extra allowance, and children's allowances will be appropriately reduced.

b) Invalidity Allowance is only paid if you start claiming more than five years before pension age, and is paid according to how old you are at the start of the claim.

c) Additional Earnings Related Pension is based on your earnings after 6 April 1978, and is paid to anyone who claims after 6 April 1979. However, the DHSS have decided that nobody can now receive *both* the Invalidity Allowance and the Additional Earnings Related in full. Further details can be found in DHSS leaflet NI 16A.

Invalidity Benefit can affect other social security benefits being claimed by either yourself or your dependants.

Invalidity Benefit is probably the most frequent benefit claimed by M.E. sufferers. You have to keep sending in sickness certificates (Med 3s) signed by your general practitioner indicating that the doctor considers that you are unfit for work. When the condition has become prolonged the general practitioner may date the certificate 'till further notice', but many GPs still like to keep an eye on their patients, and so limit it to six months or a year.

The decision to award the benefit is made by the DHSS adjudication officer – a non-medically qualified civil servant – at the local benefit office. These unnamed officials will usually accept your GP's opinion, but after a while your claim will be referred on to one of their own doctors for an opinion.

Therapeutic earnings Anyone claiming Invalidity Benefit is also allowed to have some 'therapeutic earnings' (up to £27 per week in 1988), plus a few connected expenses. You must first get written approval from your GP that the type of activity won't have any adverse effect on recovery, and then send it to the DHSS for their approval. The sort of work you might do is something quiet and non-demanding like writing, or occasionally doing your normal type of work, but for a very limited period. But, you've got to be very careful that the DHSS don't then use this activity as an excuse to say that you're fit to start looking for a full-time job again.

Invalidity Benefit cut-off The major problem that many M.E. sufferers experience in long-term sickness revolves around the DHSS definition of being 'unfit for work'. They accept that you can be off sick from your normal occupation for a certain period of time, but after that they'll only continue to pay benefit, on an indefinite basis, if they're certain that there is no other work – full-time or part-time – from which you could reasonably earn a living. For example, in the case of M.E., they might well accept that a manual worker could no longer cope with this sort of work from the physical point of view, but he could cope with something less demanding. In my case they decided I couldn't be expected to cope with making important life and death decisions when my brain wasn't functioning, but that I could do something like collecting tickets at the car park, or even be a night watchman!

The process of reviewing fitness for work is complicated. To try and explain the steps which are taken it's helpful to refer to a flow diagram.
1 The first stage is when a form arrives through the post instructing you that such a review is about to take place. This can be because either the DHSS or your GP wants a second opinion on your eligibility to benefit.
 If this happens to you – reading the impersonal, stereotyped

HOW THE SYSTEM WORKS

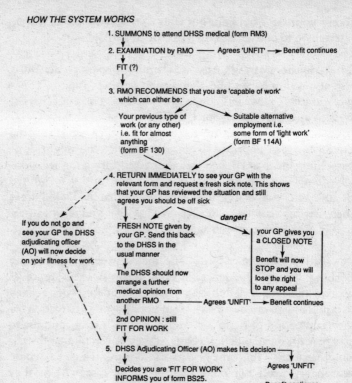

1. SUMMONS to attend DHSS medical (form RM3)

2. EXAMINATION by RMO —— Agrees 'UNFIT' → Benefit continues

   FIT (?)

3. RMO RECOMMENDS that you are 'capable of work' which can either be:

   Your previous type of work (or any other) i.e. fit for almost anything (form BF 130)

   Suitable alternative employment i.e. some form of 'light work' (form BF 114A)

4. RETURN IMMEDIATELY to see your GP with the relevant form and request a fresh sick note. This shows that your GP has reviewed the situation and still agrees you should be off sick

   If you do not go and see your GP the DHSS adjudicating officer (AO) will now decide on your fitness for work

   FRESH NOTE given by your GP. Send this back to the DHSS in the usual manner

   The DHSS should now arrange a further medical opinion from another RMO —— Agrees 'UNFIT' → Benefit continues

   2nd OPINION : still FIT FOR WORK

   danger!

   your GP gives you a CLOSED NOTE

   Benefit will now STOP and you will lose the right to any appeal

5. DHSS Adjudicating Officer (AO) makes his decision ——

   Decides you are 'FIT FOR WORK' INFORMS you of form BS25. BENEFIT WILL NOW STOP

   Agrees 'UNFIT'

   Benefit continues

6. CLAIM UNEMPLOYMENT BENEFIT
   Your GP can still issue sick notes if he disagrees.
   APPEAL within 28 days to the Social Security Appeal Tribunal (SSAT) —— → WIN APPEAL → Benefit restored and backdated

   LOSE APPEAL

7. FINAL APPEAL TO SOCIAL SECURITY COMMISSIONER

form from the DHSS telling you that your benefit has been stopped or your claim has been rejected – it's only natural to feel very angry, and even quite shocked.

Try not to get too upset, as the additional stress will only make your M.E. symptoms even worse. Sit down and calmly think things through, preferably with the help of a friend or relative for moral support, and plan what you're going to do next. Read up all the information you can get on the relevant benefit and the appeals procedures, and go and talk to someone at the local Citizens Advice Bureau. It's very tempting to start firing off a series of angry letters – by all means write them, but don't post them for forty-eight hours, as your feelings may have calmed down and changed by then. You don't want to be taking any actions in the heat of the moment which you might regret later.

When this sort of thing has happened to me, my natural reaction has been to phone the DHSS, and to try to speak to the official who's made the decision. Unfortunately, this is easier said than done, as these bureaucrats are usually well protected from members of the general public!

Where a medical decision has been taken, a form may be signed by a named divisional medical officer. These doctors aren't used to members of the public phoning them up, but if you really feel aggrieved and confident enough to do so it's well worth a try, and you may get through to the top. Again try to contain your anger, and put forward your case in a reasoned and constructive manner – you may be lucky and end up receiving some sympathetic help and advice. It's worth remembering that many of these officials and doctors don't always agree with some of the decisions they have to take when making assessments on benefit claims, and they're only too aware of defending the indefensible!

As well, go and see your GP, to find out what support (or lack of it) you're likely to get, and whether he's sent in a written report to the DHSS on your state of health. Unfortunately, some GPs are still afraid of upsetting the DHSS Regional Medical Officers (RMOs), who carry out these assessments, and don't always give their patients the support they deserve. Others, however, are excellent, and don't have any qualms about fully supporting your case, and if necessary disagreeing with a colleague's opinion.

2 The examination will take place at a local DHSS centre. If you (and your GP) can persuade the DHSS that travelling would be very difficult and harmful in your present state of health, the examining doctor might be persuaded to do the assessment at home.

The RMO is employed by the DHSS and sends an *opinion* to the local benefit office. While you're there it's worth asking if the

RMO has received a report from your GP. In some cases it may not have arrived, but they're unlikely to tell you what it says if they do have a copy.

3   The RMO has to decide if you are 'fit for work'. If it seems to him that you can't return to your normal occupation, he then has to decide if there is *any* possible work you could do. The fact that the type of work may not actually be available in your locality is of very minor consideration. Could you do it if it were available? Remember, the RMO's report is only a *recommendation*, not an arbitrary decision, although the way this information is conveyed, on Forms BF130 or BF114a, makes this far from clear.

4   If you disagree with an RMO recommendation you should immediately go and see your general practitioner and discuss the situation with him. Take the form with you as the doctor may not have heard from the DHSS. If your GP takes your side, and disagrees with the opinion – accepting you are still unfit for work – you should ask him to issue a fresh sickness certificate, even if your old one hasn't yet expired.

Your GP doesn't have to agree with the RMO – if he now issues you with a closed note (saying you are now 'fit for work') your benefit will stop, and you lose any chance of taking the case to appeal.

If the DHSS now receives your fresh certificate, they should then arrange a second medical opinion by another of their RMOs.

5   With the above medical recommendation(s) the DHSS Adjudicating Officer (AO) will now make a *decision* on the claim. The AO is a lay person, not a doctor.

6   If the AO decides to agree with the RMO the benefit will stop. However, you can now make an appeal to the Social Security Appeals Tribunal (SSAT) which consists of a lawyer and two independent people. In the meantime you do no harm by signing on as unemployed in order to get some financial help, but there's nothing to stop you sending in sickness certificates – providing your GP will still issue them. You must now prepare for the appeal by:

(a) Obtaining written support on your incapacity to work from both your GP and consultant – if you have one. The DHSS is unlikely to have obtained a consultant's report, and if this supports your claim it can be very persuasive with the tribunal.

(b) Get as much advice as possible on how to appeal from the local Citizens Advice Bureau (they might be able to send someone along with you for support), your trade union, or a disability rights organisation – e.g. the Disability Alliance.

(c) Write down a list of your symptoms and how they incapacitate you during the day, especially in ways which would affect your capacity to work – e.g. you can't be reliable as your symptoms vary so much from one day to the next.

7 If you lose this SSAT appeal you still have one last chance, by appealing to the Social Security Commissioner.

SEVERE DISABLEMENT ALLOWANCE (SDA)

For anyone who has been unable to work for twenty-eight weeks or more, but doesn't qualify for state sickness benefit or Invalidity Benefit, due to insufficient national insurance contributions. You must be aged 16–60 (women), or 16–65 (men), and get a weekly payment which is tax-free and not means-tested. There are extra additions for any adult or child dependants. You can automatically claim SDA if you already receive a Mobility or Attendance Allowance, or have an invalid car from the DHSS. You can also have 'therapeutic earnings' (see page 185). Further details on DHSS leaflet NI 252.

You must be both incapable of work, *and* be assessed as being 75 per cent or more disabled.

Assessing a percentage disability for say loss of a limb is relatively straightforward, but with M.E., where the disability is fluctuating and hard to assess objectively, it's quite likely that different doctors will come to differing conclusions. You'll almost certainly have to go for a medical examination, and if your general practitioner or consultant is prepared to support your case, it's important to make sure they send in some written evidence to this effect, clearly stating the nature of the disabilities M.E. is causing. The assessment should take into account both your physical and mental disabilities associated with M.E., and how they are preventing you carrying out 'normal living', with particular reference to employment prospects.

In the case of M.E. the disabilities which are particularly relevant are:

- Limited energy, which affects your ability to walk or carry out physical tasks.
- Brain malfunction, affecting your mental abilities.

It's important to get these facts clear in your mind before you go to the examination, so you can present them to the examining doctors when they question you about how M.E. affects your life.

SDA is a very complex benefit in its qualifying criteria, and so before making an application I'd recommend any sufferer to read more about it in the *Disability Rights Handbook*. More specific information is contained in – *The SDA – Handbook for Adjudicating Medical Authorities*, price £1 from the DHSS leaflets unit (see page 202).

If you apply and are then refused you do have a right to appeal – within three months – to a Medical Appeal Tribunal. From talking to M.E. sufferers who've been refused on their first attempt, my advice is to appeal, and if still unsuccessful to try again at a later date. Unfortunately, one doctor's view of disability isn't always the same as his colleagues'.

ATTENDANCE ALLOWANCE

This is for people who are *severely disabled*, and need a lot of looking after. Living alone is not a disqualification. Anyone aged two or over is eligible. There's no upper age limit, but you have to fulfil the qualifying criteria for six months before a claim can be accepted. (You can apply before this six-month qualifying period, though.)

There is a weekly payment at two rates: a low rate, for either daytime or night-time care, and a high rate, for both daytime and night-time care. Attendance Allowance is not means-tested or taxable, and you don't have to have made any national insurance contributions. If you make a successful claim for AA, then the person who is looking after you may qualify for Invalid Care Allowance. Claim on form NI 205.

This isn't an allowance which is likely to benefit many M.E.

sufferers as it's primarily aimed at people who continually require a lot of help and attention with what the DHSS refers to as 'bodily functions'. By this, they mean assistance from other people with walking, dressing, washing, eating, and going to the toilet, etc. Anyone who thinks that they may be eligible should read more about Attendance Allowance in the *Disability Rights Handbook*.

If you apply, the DHSS will then arrange for a medical examination, which is carried out at your home. The doctor's report will then go to an Attendance Allowance Board, where another doctor will make the actual decision. You'll then receive a certificate giving you the allowance, with a time limit on it, after which a further review will be necessary. However, there's still one further hurdle. You also have to be passed as eligible by a DHSS adjudication officer on the non-medical aspects of the claim.

If your claim is refused there are appeal procedures which can be followed. Appeals on non-medical grounds go to the Social Security Appeals Tribunal, or, if you've been turned down on medical grounds, you can ask the Board's doctor to review the case. If you decide to appeal it's essential to take expert advice on how to prepare for such an appeal, and again follow the advice in the *Disability Rights Handbook*.

THE INVALID CARE ALLOWANCE

This is for people of working age (16–60 for women, and 16–65 for men) who can't go out to work because they're having to look after someone at home who is severely disabled, i.e., obtaining the Attendance Allowance. National insurance contributions are not required, but the payment is taxable. There are additions for dependent relatives, but it can be affected by other social security benefits. Claim on form NI 212.

To qualify for ICA you must be spending thirty-five hours or more in 'caring'; any earnings above £12 per week may affect this benefit. You don't, however, have to be related to the person you're looking after.

If a claim for ICA is refused, you can appeal to the Social Security Appeals Tribunal.

HOME RESPONSIBILITIES PROTECTION

If you're not eligible for Invalid Care Allowance, but still having to stay at home to look after a severely disabled person you may qualify for this. If you're claiming certain other social security benefits you may already be having your national insurance contributions credited by the DHSS, and so protecting pension rights. If this isn't the case then you should check with the DHSS if you ought to apply for HRP.

The *Disability Rights Handbook* also covers the benefit in detail.

MOBILITY ALLOWANCE

An allowance for patients who are unable or virtually unable to walk, and likely to remain so for at least one year. It is available to ages 5–66, but once awarded can continue till you are 75. It is tax free, not means-tested, and you claim on DHSS form 211. It acts as a passport to various other benefits: British Rail disabled railcard, car tax exemption, orange parking badge.

Mobility Allowance, in theory, is just the sort of benefit which ought to be of great value to M.E. sufferers who are having to rely on public transport. You can spend the benefit any way you wish to improve mobility – taxi fares, or towards a new car, etc. Unfortunately, in practice, very few M.E. sufferers are currently receiving it, although the success rate does seem to be steadily increasing. The reasons for this difficulty are threefold. First, the qualifying criteria are interpreted very strictly, and the DHSS may be worried about the increasing number of people with all types of illness receiving MA, along with the fact that it's not always being used to increase their mobility. Second, some of the examining doctors are still very sceptical about the degree of muscular fatigue and weakness that M.E. causes. Third, even if the doctor accepts the diagnosis of M.E., they don't like making awards if a condition seems to be fluctuating in severity.

In order to qualify you have to demonstrate that your muscular weakness will satisfy one of three definitions:

(a) Being completely unable to walk. This means that you can't take a single step, and very few M.E. sufferers fall into this category.

(b) Being virtually unable to walk. Here the DHSS are not terribly specific in terms of distance; however, anyone who is capable of walking unaided for more than a few hundred yards seems unlikely to qualify. Your walking ability does have to be considerably restricted.

(c) The exertion required to walk constitutes either a danger to life, or could lead to a serious deterioration in health. Again, the interpretation is far from clear when it comes to M.E. Those sufferers who have very severe limitations in their exercise capabilities before becoming exhausted may well find that they fulfil this part of the criteria.

The only way to find out if you can get a Mobility Allowance is to fill in the claim form and see what happens. The DHSS will then arrange a medical examination, often by a general practitioner who frequently does such assessments. The examination is usually arranged at a surgery, but can be at your home if necessary. (You can also request to be examined by a lady doctor.) The doctor's report will then be sent to the DHSS adjudicating officer (a non-medically qualified civil servant) who decides on the claim. If there is still any doubt you then have to be seen by a medical board, at the nearest DHSS Medical Examination Centre, before the adjudicating officer makes a decision.

If you're refused, you can appeal (within three months), and then you must organise written support from anyone who you think might help, e.g. your general practitioner, consultant or physiotherapist. This written support must state very clearly the exact nature of your walking disabilities, and the weakness or fatigue caused by M.E. Your appeal against either the original doctor's report, or the medical board's ruling will be heard by a Medical Appeal Tribunal. Once the tribunal has made its decision there is no further right of appeal, but there's nothing to stop you making a further application after a reasonable period of time if you feel that problems are no better, or have got worse.

It may take some perseverance to get a Mobility Allowance, including going through these appeal procedures, but don't give up if you think you have a strong case. If you feel really aggrieved by a refusal you can still write to your MP and ask him to put your case to the Secretary of State for Social Services.

SOME OF YOUR 'RIGHTS' FROM THE NHS

You don't have many 'rights' from the NHS – just reasonable requests.

Home visits You can't demand to have your GP visit you at home – it's up to your doctor's individual judgement, depending on your symptoms at the time. Doctors are becoming more reluctant to do home visiting for the chronic sick, and prefer you to come to the surgery whenever possible. However, your doctor is obliged, under his contract, to come out and visit in an emergency.

Drugs Again, you can't demand to have a new treatment which you may have heard about, but which your GP isn't yet aware of. Doctors are quite rightly reluctant to start prescribing new drugs until their benefits have been proved and long-term side-effects fully established. If your GP is unfamiliar with the use of a drug in M.E. such as the gammaglobulin injections, he'll probably want to discuss this with a specialist before giving it. It seems that long legal actions against doctors, for side-effects from drugs they've prescribed, are going to be increasingly common, so such caution will very likely increase.

Second opinions Patients don't have any 'right' to a second opinion from a specialist, but it would be unreasonable if a GP refused such a request when there were doubts about either the diagnosis, or how the illness should be managed. Under the NHS you can't choose which specialist you want to be referred to, but there's nothing to stop you suggesting a particular name if you've heard that this consultant is sympathetic to or interested in M.E.

Complaints about doctors If you want to make a complaint about your medical treatment from a GP it has to be done within eight weeks of whatever incident prompted the complaint. This has to be made to your local Family Practitioner Committee. Complaints about medical treatment in hospital are dealt with by Regional Medical Officers. In either case your local Community Health Council will give further help and advice as to whether it would be wise to proceed.

Your medical records You don't have any 'right' to examine your medical notes kept either by the hospital or your GP. These notes are officially the property of the Secretary of State for Health. Some M.E. patients get very annoyed, quite rightly, when inaccurate opinions about their illness get into their notes, and it then seems almost impossible to get such statements removed. If you feel really strongly about this there are procedures that can be followed, and again the local Community Health Council should be able to help. Some doctors are becoming increasingly willing for their patients to see their own notes (in France patients carry their own notes around with them), but most remain firmly opposed to such 'freedom of information' for their patients.

MISCELLANEOUS FINANCIAL PROBLEMS

Private health insurance (sick pay) schemes Just as the DHSS may decide to stop paying Invalidity Benefit on the grounds that you could find 'suitable alternative employment', you may also find that if you're covered by a private sick pay insurance scheme, the same sort of terminology is being used after a similar period of time. Check the small print.

Life insurance and M.E. This is one other piece of financial planning which occasionally causes difficulty. Most of the large insurance companies won't refuse M.E. sufferers life insurance, although the cost of the policy might be slightly loaded.

M.E. is not a life-threatening condition, and most companies readily accept this, although you may have to 'shop around' or go to a broker who is experienced in dealing with clients who have health difficulties for a competitive quote.

2. Useful Names And Addresses

THE M.E. ASSOCIATION

This is a particularly important source of practical advice, help and support. It is a self-help group, formed in 1976, which now has well over 10,000 members. Dr Melvin Ramsay is its President.

The Association is run by a central committee of volunteers, and organised into a large number of locally based groups. These local groups are starting to cover most of the country, and exist in most large towns, or counties covering rural areas. As they become established they're starting to hold regular meetings throughout the year, and arranging guest speakers. There are also full-time paid employees at the office in Essex, who deal with an ever mounting number of queries and letters arriving each day (sometimes over 1,000 after a piece of television publicity) from patients, doctors, journalists – in fact anyone wanting to know more about M.E.

The Association tries to help with all aspects of M.E., ranging from advice on welfare problems, through to raising money for the various medical research projects. An Annual General Meeting is held in London, usually in mid-April, and the 1988 meeting attracted well over 1,000 doctors and patients, some even travelling long distances from abroad. This annual meeting is an all-day event, and well worth attending if you can possibly get there. There are medical talks and discussions with the specialists involved in M.E. research at the university hospitals, as well as smaller sessions devoted to other aspects of living with M.E. Most patients go away better informed about the illness than their own doctors! The Association also has a group of doctors expert in M.E., who act as medical advisors, and can help with specific queries from other members of the medical profession.

Trying to make sure that M.E. receives positive publicity in the media is another important function for the Association, and this includes persuading journalists not to sensationalise or dismiss the subject. Part of this publicity and awareness process also involves contact with Members of Parliament and DHSS ministers, to make sure the disease is accepted as a genuine physical illness (which they now concede), and making sure that sufferers are receiving a fair deal when it comes to obtaining sickness and other disability benefits.

Last, the Association tries hard to look after members' welfare and emotional difficulties. Help can be offered if there is a hassle with benefits or problems with employment. A 'listening ear' service run by volunteers is another valuable service which enables any member to ring up and have a chat or discuss a problem with someone else who's not only understanding and knows about M.E., but may also be able to offer some practical solutions. Special groups also operate for single members, those who are looking after children and have M.E., patients for whom religious faith is important, and young people.

Membership currently costs £8 per year. For full details send a stamped addressed envelope to the

> M.E. Association
> PO Box 8
> Stanford le Hope,
> Essex SS17 8EX.

Abroad, self-help groups are also operating in:

Australia: M.E. Society
                  PO Box 645
                  Mona Vale, NSW, 2103

New Zealand: PO Box 35/429
                  Browns Bay
                  Auckland 10

Canada: Mrs K. M. Smith
                  PO Box 298
                  Kleinburg
                  Ontario, L0J 1C0

Holland: Ms Marion Lescrauwaet
                    1106 DP Wamelplein 16
                    Amsterdam
Irish Republic: Ms Miriam Sheridan
                    80 Foxfield Road
                    Raheny
                    Dublin 5
Norway: Ms Ellen Piro (Norges M.E. Forening)
                    Gullerasveien 14B
                    0386 Oslo 3
South Africa: Mrs Janine Shavell
                    66 Third Street
                    Lower-Houghton
                    Johannesburg

More groups are currently being planned in other parts of the world as well.

THE M.E. ACTION CAMPAIGN

The M.E. Action Campaign is a pressure group campaigning on a variety of issues connected with M.E. and has Clare Francis – a fellow sufferer – as President.

The Action Campaign has used the media and lobbied Members of Parliament and the DHSS to fully recognise the illness, and provide more funds for vital research. It was recently successful in persuading Jimmy Hood, MP for Clydesdale, to introduce a Bill in the House of Commons (*Hansard*, 23 February 1988: pages 167–8) to draw attention to the multitude of problems which M.E. sufferers face. The Bill received wide all-party support, which was probably helped by the fact that there are members in both houses with M.E.

The Action Campaign feels that research into the condition needs to be particularly directed at the reasons why some people are more susceptible to these viruses, and why they go on to persist in the body. They're also interested in exploring and researching a wide range of treatments which appear to help (e.g. dietary modification, identification of allergies and sensitivities, and anti-candida treatment), whether or not they have the approval of conventional medical opinion.

The Campaign isn't a membership organisation. It will provide information on its activities and ideas on request. Above all, it feels that sufferers need to take responsibility for their own health, and take whatever action is necessary to promote a return to well-being. For further information, send a stamped addressed envelope to:

> M.E. Action Campaign
> PO Box 1126
> London W3 0RY

GENERAL ADDRESSES, A–Z

Acupuncture

MEDICALLY QUALIFIED ACUPUNCTURISTS
British Medical Acupuncture Society
67–69 Chancery Lane
London WC2 1AF

NON-MEDICALLY QUALIFIED
ACUPUNCTURISTS
British Acupuncture Association
34 Alderney Street
London SW1B 4EU

CHINESE DOCTORS PRACTISING
ACUPUNCTURE
Chinese Medical Association
59 Cumberland Place
London W1

ADVISORY CENTRE FOR EDUCATION
18 Victoria Park Square
London E2 9PB
Tel (01) 980 4596

ALTERNATIVE MEDICINE
Institute for Complementary Medicine
21 Portland Place
London WC1N 3AF

ASSOCIATION OF CARERS
First Floor
21–23 New Road
Chatham
Kent ME4 4QJ
Tel (0634) 813981

ASSOCIATION OF SWIMMING THERAPY
Mr Ted Cowen (Secretary)
4 Oak Street
Shrewsbury SY3 7RH
Tel (0743) 4393
(Publishes *Swimming for the Disabled*)

BACK PAIN ASSOCIATION
31–33 Park Road
Teddington
Middlesex TW11 0AB
Tel (01) 977 5474
Free leaflets (send SAE) and cassettes available

BRITISH ASSOCIATION OF COUNSELLING
37A Sheep Street
Rugby
Warwickshire CV21 3BX
Tel (0788) 78328
Publishes directories of counsellors, as well as helping with
psychosexual problems

BRITISH HOLISTIC MEDICAL ASSOCIATION
179 Gloucester Place
London NW1 6DX
Tel (01) 262 5299
Lists of medically qualified practitioners of holistic medicine.
Leaflets on therapies and cassettes. Runs relaxation and medi-
tation classes. Twenty-eight branches nationwide (five in Lon-
don)

BRITISH RED CROSS SOCIETY
9 Grosvenor Crescent
London SW1X 7EJ
Tel (01) 235 5454
Local branches are listed in the phone book

BRITISH SPORTS ASSOCIATION FOR THE
DISABLED
Hayward House
Barnard Crescent
Aylesbury
Bucks HP21 9PP
Tel (0296) 27889
Encouragement and advice on all forms of sporting activities for
the disabled

CAPITAL RADIO HELPLINE
Euston Tower
London NW1 3DR
Tel (01) 388 7575
A confidential off-air advice and information service for people
in London. Experienced counsellors will try to advise on any
sort of problem, or put you in touch with a relevant organisation
who could help

CENTRE ON THE ENVIRONMENT FOR THE
HANDICAPPED
35 Great Smith Street
London SW1P 3BJ
Tel (01) 222 7980
An organisation concerned with the physical environment of
disabled people. Can help with architectural design of building
adaptations

CHILDREN IN HOSPITAL (National Association for the
Welfare of)
Argyle House
29–31 Euston Road
London NW1 2SD
Tel (01) 833 2041

CHIROPRACTIC – BRITISH CHIROPRACTORS' ASSOCIATION
5 First Avenue
Chelmsford
Essex CM1 1RX
Tel (0245) 358487

CHRONIC FATIGUE & IMMUNE DEFICIENCY SOCIETY (CEBV SYNDROME)
PO Box 230108
Portland
Oregon 97223
USA
Information on CEBV, and newsletter available

COLLEGE OF HEALTH
18 Victoria Park Square
London E2 9PF
Tel (01) 980 6263
Aims to improve self-care and self-help groups through proper use of the NHS and alternative therapies. Publishes a wide range of useful leaflets. HEALTHLINE service has over 200 tapes which can be heard over the phone – Tel (01) 980 4848 from 2–10 p.m. daily. Full directory available by post. Also publishes the journal *Self-Health* which covers both orthodox and alternative medicine

CROSSROADS CARE ATTENDANT SCHEMES
94 Coton Road
Rugby
Warwickshire CV21 4LN
Tel (0788) 73653
Help in the home for disabled people and locally based groups

DHSS
Leaflets from Leaflets Unit
PO Box 21
Stanmore
Middlesex HA7 1AY
Freephone advice line (0800) 666555 (often engaged) gives free advice on DHSS benefits

DISABLEMENT INFORMATION AND ADVICE LINES (DIAL)
Victoria Buildings
117 High Street
Clay Cross
Derbyshire S45 9DZ
Tel (0246) 864498
Free confidential information and advice on a wide variety of issues concerning disabled people. Eighty branches throughout the U.K.

DISABILITY ALLIANCE
25 Denmark Street
London WC2H 8NJ
Tel (01) 240 0806
Pressure group which campaigns on benefits for the disabled. Publishes the *Disability Rights Handbook*, an invaluable guide through the DHSS benefit maze. Also does research into financial problems of disability

DISABLED DRIVERS' ASSOCIATION
Drake House
18 Creekside
London SE8 3DZ
Tel (01) 692 7141
Information and advice for disabled drivers

DISABLED DRIVERS' MOTOR CLUB
1a Dudley Gardens
London W13 9LU
Tel (01) 840 1515
Helps with cross-Channel ferry concessions, and promotes the interests of physically disabled drivers

DISABLEMENT INCOME GROUP (DIG)
Attlee House
28 Commercial Street
London E1 6LR
Tel (01) 247 2128/6877
Operates advisory service on benefits. Several publications – list on request. Nineteen local branches – see phone book

DISABLED LIVING FOUNDATION
380–384 Harrow Road
London W9 2HU
Tel (01) 289 6111
Information and advice on a huge number of aids for the
disabled. Exhibitions open in local centres but appointment is
necessary

Local centres in:

Belfast	Tel (0232) 669501
Birmingham	(021) 643 0980
Blackpool	(0253) 21084
Caerphilly	(0222) 887325
Cardiff	(0222) 566281
Dudley	(0384) 237034
Edinburgh	(031) 447 6271
Huddersfield	(0484) 518809
Leeds	(0532) 793140
Leicester	(0533) 700747
Liverpool	(051) 228 9221
London	(01) 289 6111
Macclesfield	(0625) 21000
Manchester	(061) 832 3678
Middlesbrough	(0642) 813133
Newcastle	(091) 2840480
Paisley	(041) 887 0597
Portsmouth	(0705) 737174
Sheffield	(0742) 737025
Southampton	(0703) 777222
Stockport	(061) 419 4476
Swindon	(0793) 643966

EQUIPMENT FOR THE DISABLED
Mary Marlborough Lodge
Nuffield Orthopaedic Centre
Headington
Oxford OX3 7LD
Tel (0865) 750103
Publishes a series of useful illustrated booklets on various aspects

of disability (e.g. wheelchairs, disabled mothers) each acting as a reference source

FAMILY WELFARE ASSOCIATION
501–505 Kingsland Road
London E8 4AU
Tel (01) 254 6251
Professional counselling service for families in distress. Ten local branches in the U.K.

HEALING – CHURCHES COUNCIL FOR HEALTH AND HEALING
St Marylebone Parish Church
Marylebone Road
London NW1 5LT
Tel (01) 486 9644
An interdenominational organisation which can answer enquiries concerning religion and medicine, and information on healing services

NATIONAL FEDERATION OF SPIRITUAL HEALING
Old Manor Farm Studio
Church Street
Sunbury on Thames
Middlesex

HERBALISTS – THE BRITISH HERBAL MEDICINE ASSOCIATION
3 Amberwood House
Walkford
Dorset BN23 5RT
Runs an information service and a list of herbal practitioners. Medically-qualified herbalists have been trained by the National Institute for Medical Herbalists

BRITISH HOLISTIC MEDICAL ASSOCIATION
179 Gloucester Place
London NW1
Tel (01) 262 5299

Homeopathy

BRITISH HOMEOPATHIC ASSOCIATION
27a Devonshire Street
London W1N 1RJ
Tel (01) 935 2163
Any doctor who has completed a recognised course in homeopathy has the letters MFHom after his name

SOCIETY OF HOMEOPATHS
47 Canada Grove
Bognor Regis
Sussex PO21 1DD
Tel (0243) 860678
Society of non-medically qualified homeopaths. Members have the letters RSHom after their names

HOMEOPATHIC HOSPITALS
Found in: Bristol
        Glasgow
        Liverpool
        London
        Tunbridge Wells
For more information, send SAE to:
The Faculty of Homeopathy
The Royal Homeopathic Hospital
Great Ormond Street
London WC1N 3HR

HOMEOPATHIC MEDICINES
Ainsworths Homeopathic Pharmacy
38 New Cavendish Street
London W1M 7LH
Tel (01) 935 5330
They can be prescribed on the NHS, but are not too expensive to purchase in general

HYPNOSIS
The British Society of Medical and Dental Hypnosis
42 Links Road
Ashtead
Surrey
Tel (0372) 73522

INVALID CHILDREN'S AID ASSOCIATION
126 Buckingham Palace Road
London SW1W 9SB
Tel (01) 730 9891
Help and advice for parents with problems associated with
disabled children – will advise on educational difficulties

LONDON DIAL-A-RIDE
St Margarets
25 Leighton Road
London NW5 2QD
Tel (01) 482 2325
Information on London Dial-a-Ride services

LONDON TAXICARD
Apply at any large post office

MARRIAGE GUIDANCE COUNCIL (RELATE)
Herbert Gray College
Little Church
Rugby
Warks CV21 3AP
Tel (0788) 73241
Local branches in the phone book

M.E. ASSOCIATION
See beginning of this chapter

M.E. ACTION CAMPAIGN
See beginning of this chapter

MEDIC-ALERT FOUNDATION
11–13 Clifton Terrace
London N4 3JP
Tel (01) 263 8596
Produces bracelets/medallions with twenty-four-hour tele-

phone number of their office, which keeps details of your medical condition

MIND (National Association for Mental Health)
22 Harley Street
London W1N 2ED
Tel (01) 637 0741
Campaigning group on a range of issues to do with mental health. Publishes booklets and leaflets on a variety of issues concerned with psychiatric illness. Has a legal department which will help with any mental health problem which requires this sort of advice, e.g. discharge from a psychiatric hospital. Two hundred local groups – see the phone book

MOBILITY ADVICE AND VEHICLE INFORMATION SERVICES (MAVIS)
Department of Transport
Transport and Road Research Laboratory
Crowthorne
Berkshire RG11 6AU
Tel (0344) 779014

MOTABILITY
2nd Floor
Gate House
Westgate
The High
Harlow
Essex CM20 1HR
Tel (0279) 635666
Helps people in receipt of Mobility Allowance get the best value for money including hire purchase of cars and wheelchairs, and a car leasing scheme

NATIONAL ASSOCIATION FOR PRE-MENSTRUAL SYNDROME
25 Market Street
Guildford
Surrey GU1 4LB
Tel (0483) 572715
Self-help group for sufferers

NATUROPATHY – THE BRITISH NATUROPATHIC AND OSTEOPATHIC ASSOCIATION
Frazer House
6 Netherall Gardens
London NW3 5RR
Tel (01) 435 8728
Members use the initials ND, DO or MBNOA after a four-year training, but do not advertise

OCCUPATIONAL PENSIONS ADVISORY SERVICE
Room 327
Aviation House
129 Kingsway
London WC2B 6NN
Tel (01) 379 7311, ext 6205

OPEN UNIVERSITY
Adviser on the Education of Disabled Students
Walton Hall
Milton Keynes MK7 6AA
Home study and courses suitable for disabled students

OPPORTUNITIES FOR THE DISABLED
1 Bank Buildings
Princes Street
London EC2R 8EU
Tel (01) 726 4961
Employment service for job seekers and employers. Eleven regional offices

OSTEOPATHY – THE GENERAL COUNCIL AND REGISTER OF OSTEOPATHS
1 Suffolk Street
London SW1
Tel (01) 839 2060
Keeps a list of qualified osteopaths

PAIN RELIEF CLINICS
The Honourable Secretary
Intractable Pain Society of Great Britain and Ireland
Basingstoke District Hospital
Hants

Locations of local pain relief centres

PATIENTS' ASSOCIATION
Room 33
18 Charing Cross Road
London WC2H 0HR
Tel (01) 240 0671
Help and advice to patients on any aspect of health care. Can help in resolving complaints against doctors and hospitals. Campaigns for better monitoring of drugs and their side-effects, and allowing patients to see their own medical records

PHOBIC ACTION
Greater London House
547–551 High Road
Leytonstone
London E11 4PR
Tel (01) 558 6012
Help for phobia sufferers in London

PHOBIC SOCIETY
4 Cheltenham Road
Chorlton-cum-Hardy
Manchester M21 1QN
Tel (061) 881 1937
Help, advice and information on phobias. Network of nine local branches

PHYSIOTHERAPISTS
Mrs M. Briggs
50 Mannering Gardens
Westcliff-on-Sea
Essex SS0 0BQ
Produces a directory of chartered physiotherapists working in private practice

RADAR (ROYAL ASSOCIATION FOR DISABILITY AND REHABILITATION)
25 Mortimer Street
London W1N 8AB
Tel (01) 637 5400

Umbrella organisation giving advice on all matters related to disability: access, holidays (publishes useful guides), housing, mobility, welfare and employment. Large number of publications and leaflets

RAYNAUD'S ASSOCIATION TRUST
40 Bladon Crescent
Alsager
Cheshire ST7 2BG
Tel (09363) 5167
Information, newsletters and practical advice on Raynaud's syndrome (cold hands and feet)

REHABILITATION ENGINEERING MOVEMENT
ADVISORY PANEL
25 Mortimer Street
London W1N 8AB
Tel (01) 637 5400
Panel of engineers, doctors and therapists who try to provide practical solutions to the problems of disability

RELAXATION FOR LIVING
29 Burwood Park Road
Walton-on-Thames
Surrey KT12 5LH
Information on relaxation techniques, and courses: send large SAE

SAMARITANS
17 Uxbridge Road
Slough
Berkshire LS1 1SN
Tel (0753) 32713/4
About 180 local branches (see phone book) giving a confidential service over the phone for anyone in despair

SOCIAL SECURITY COMMISSIONERS
Harp House
83 Farringdon Street
London EC4A 4BT
Final appeals on benefit refusals

SOCIETY FOR HORTICULTURAL THERAPY
Goulds Ground
Vallis Way
Frome
Somerset BA11 3DW
Tel (0373) 64782
Promotes gardening as a form of therapy for people with disabilities

SPOD (ASSOCIATION TO AID SEXUAL AND PERSONAL RELATIONSHIPS OF PEOPLE WITH A DISABILITY)
286 Camden Road
London N7 0BJ
Tel (01) 607 8851/2
Information and advice on sexuality and disability. Can put patients in touch with experienced sexual counsellors. Also publishes leaflets and information

TINNITUS ASSOCIATION
c/o Royal National Institute for the Deaf
105 Gower Street
London WC1E 6AH
Tel (01) 387 8033

TRANX UK (NATIONAL TRANQUILLISER ADVISORY COUNCIL)
17 Peel Road
Harrow
Middlesex HA3 7QX
Tel (01) 427 2065
Advice and support for people using tranquillisers on a long-term basis – and help to get off them

YOUTHLINE
54 Hamlet Road
Southend-on-Sea
Essex SS1 1HH
Tel (0702) 340804
Confidential telephone service for young people to talk over their problems. Part of the Samaritans

3. Further Reading

HOW TO OBTAIN MEDICAL REFERENCES

References from medical journals are from publications which shouldn't be too hard to find in a medical library. There's no 'embargo' on the general public obtaining this sort of information if they decide to do so. Many doctors are very opposed to patients reading scientific literature of this type, as they feel (with some justification) that patients get the wrong ideas and misinterpret symptoms and management advice. And, a few of them don't actually like the idea of their patients knowing more about a condition than they do!

If you want to get a photocopy of a reference, phone your local public library librarian, and ask if they'll do this for you – they're usually very obliging, even finding references which are quite obscure. You'll have to pay a small fee, but it shouldn't cost too much.

Unfortunately, if you go to a medical library and try to look up M.E. in one of the large medical textbooks, you still won't find very much of use, and sometimes nothing at all. I recently surveyed a large number of new editions of standard medical textbooks on infectious diseases and neurology. The results were dismaying. Even the latest edition of probably the most influential textbook on infectious diseases in the U.K. failed to even mention M.E. As a result I'm now in the process of tackling individual editors of these reference books to try and persuade them to include accurate accounts in their next editions. If your own doctor says he can't find anything about M.E. in his books, this is the reason why!

RESEARCH INTO MYALGIC ENCEPHALOMYELITIS

These are the sort of references which your doctor ought to be reading if he's become interested in the subject and wants to learn more. You may also want to find out more yourself.

Dr Peter Behan's comprehensive research study on fifty patients was published in the *Journal of Infection* (October 1985: 10; pp. 211–22).

Professor Radda's nuclear magnetic resonance findings were published in *The Lancet* (23 June 1984: pp. 1367–9).

The Scottish outbreaks of M.E. during the 1980s have been recorded in various issues of the *Journal of the Royal College of General Practitioners* including:

1983: 33; pp. 339–41 and pp. 335–7
1984: 34; pp. 3–6 and pp. 15–19
1987: 37; pp. 11–14.

Professor James Mowbray's results on testing for persisting enteroviral infection appear in *The Lancet* (23 January 1988: pp. 146–50), and this includes the 'VP1 test'.

A very comprehensive account of enteroviral infections in general, by Dr Betty Dowsett, was published in the *Journal of Hospital Infection* (1988: 11; pp. 103–15).

The Australian findings on red blood cell abnormalities were also published in *The Lancet* (8 August 1987: pp. 328–9).

Dr Melvin Ramsay's book *Myalgic Encephalomyelitis and Post Viral Fatigue States* also covers the progress in research into M.E. right from the first recorded outbreak in 1934. It is available from the M.E. Association.

Doctors McEvedy and Beard's papers (concluding that the mass Royal Free outbreak was hysteria) appeared in the *British Medical Journal* in January 1970 (1; pp. 7–11 and pp. 11–15). The reasons why their findings are now so critically refuted are discussed in Dr Melvin Ramsay's book.

A very useful book on how to make the best use of doctors and the National Health Service – *Consumer's Guide to Health Information* – is available from the College of Health, 18 Victoria Park Square, London E2 9PF, price £3.95.

A Year Lost and Found recounts the experiences of Michael

Mayne, Dean of Westminster, a fellow sufferer from M.E.; it's available from Darton, Longman & Todd Ltd, 89 Lillie Road, London SW6 1UD. Michael Mayne has recently agreed to become Vice President of the M.E. Association.

THE WORLDWIDE INCIDENCE OF M.E.

Very readable accounts of the recent Lake Tahoe outbreak in America appeared in the U.S. magazines *Hippocrates* (July 1987) and *Rolling Stone* (16 July and 13 August 1987).

The link between Epstein-Barr virus is discussed in a *Lancet* editorial, 4 May 1985: pp. 1017–18.

Recent scientific findings from America in relation to Epstein-Barr virus are contained in several articles in the *Journal of the American Medical Association*, 1 May 1987.

Dr Stephen Straus, who maintains a keen interest in the subject of post-viral fatigue has written a very comprehensive review of the subject – as viewed from the other side of the Atlantic – in the *Journal of Infectious Diseases*, March 1988, pp. 405–12.

SECONDARY PROBLEMS

Anxiety
Understanding Stress is published by *Which*, and is available from the Consumers Association (14 Buckingham Street, London WC2).

Claire Weekes has also written a book which many people find helpful – *Self-help for your Nerves* (Angus & Robertson, 1981).

Depression
Dealing with Depression by Kathy Nairne and Gerrilyn Smith (Women's Press, 1984).
Depression, The Way Out of Your Prison by Dorothy Rowe (Routledge & Kegan Paul, 1983).

Tranquilliser abuse

Dr Vernon Coleman's book *Life Without Tranquillisers* (Corgi, 1986) describes this problem in detail, and gives information for both doctors and patients on how to come off these drugs.

For carers

Caring at Home by Nancy Kohner, published by the National Extension College, Cambridge. Essential reading for any carer – packed with useful information.

ALTERNATIVE APPROACHES

General

The Handbook of Complementary Medicine by Stephen Fulder (Coronet, 1984) is a useful reference book giving detailed accounts of fifteen different therapies.

The College of Health Guide to Alternative Medicine is a similar but shorter guide. Available direct from the College of Health (see Useful Addresses).

Clinical Ecology: The Treatment of Ill Health Caused by Environmental Factors by Drs George Lewith and Julian Kenyon (Thorsons, 1985) is a useful study of the effects of the environment on health.

Acupuncture

Alternative Therapies by G. T. Lewith (Heinemann Medical, 1985).

Acupuncture, The Ancient Chinese Art of Healing and How It Works Scientifically by F. Mann (Heinemann Medical, 1982).

Candida albicans

The Yeast Connection by Dr William Crook MD (Random House UK, 1988) describes the alternative view on candida and its alleged role in health and disease.

Herbal medicines

The Drug and Therapeutics Bulletin (15 December 1986) is a publication for doctors: it carried an excellent review of both the benefits and possible side-effects from herbal medicines.

Information on individual herbs can be found in:

British Herbal Pharmacopoeia, published in three volumes by the British Herbal Medicine Association, London, a scientific committee of herbalists, pharmacologists, pharmacists and doctors. It's very comprehensive.

The Encyclopedia of Herbs and Herbalism by M. Stuart (Orbis, 1979) gives medicinal uses of 400-plus herbs.

Mary Grieve's *A Modern Herbal* (Penguin, 1977) combines ancient and traditional folklore on the subject, as well as botanical descriptions, medicinal usage and dosage.

Homeopathy

Introduction to Homeopathic Medicine by H. Boyd (Beaconsfield, 1981).

Relaxation

Breath of Life – Undoing Muscular Tension is a tape produced by the British Holistic Medical Association (see Useful Addresses), which some patients have found helpful.

PRACTICAL AIDS

The *British Medical Journal* 1988 carried a series of detailed articles covering various practical aids for the disabled:

23 January	'Collars and Corsets', p. 276
6 February	'Surgical Stockings', pp. 413–14
20 February	'Special Footwear', pp. 548–50
27 February	'Wheelchairs', pp. 625–6
5 March	'Choosing Chairs for the Disabled', pp. 701–2
12 March	'Aids for Urinary Incontinence', pp. 772–3
26 March	'Toilet Aids', pp. 918–19
2 April	'Equipment for Bathing', pp. 982–3
9 April	'Disabled Living Centres', pp. 1052–3
16 April	'Hoists', pp. 1114–17
7 May	'Provision of Aids', pp. 1317–18

These are a really useful series of articles containing information which is otherwise difficult to find. For a small fee your local public library may be quite willing to obtain photocopies. The

BMJ is published by the British Medical Association, Tavistock Square, London WC1H 9JR.

INCREASING MOBILITY

The Department of Transport (see Useful Addresses) publish an excellent *free* guide called *Door to Door* (new edition in summer 1988) giving further information on all mobility problems.

Wheelchairs The May 1988 M.E. Association Newsletter included a very helpful article on an M.E. sufferer's experiences with a wheelchair.

HOLIDAYS

RADAR (see Useful Addresses) publish useful holiday guides for disabled people:
Holidays and Travel Abroad, £1.50p from RADAR.
Holidays for Disabled People (published annually), £3.00 from bookshops or direct from RADAR.

DHSS BENEFITS

The most useful publication on DHSS benefits is
Disability Rights Handbook (published each April), £3.50 post free from the Disability Alliance (see Useful Addresses).
Also from the Disability Alliance:
Guide to Benefits for Children with Disabilities and Their Families (1988)
Attendance Allowance – Going for a Review (75p)
Mobility Allowance – Guide and Checklist (£1)
Invalid Procedures? A Study of the Control System for Invalidity Benefit (£1.30)
A Right to Work – Disability and Employment (£2)

The S.D.A. – Handbook for Adjudicating Medical Authorities, £1.00 from the DHSS leaflets unit.

INDEX

Index compiled by Peva Keane

A Full List of Cedar Books
DIRECT ORDER FORM

☐	434 11163 5	**When Am I Going to be Happy?:**	Dr Penelope Russianoff	£4.99
		How to Break the Emotional Bad Habits		
		That Make you Miserable		
☐	434 11156 2	**Living With M.E.: A Self-help Guide**	Dr Charles Shepherd	£4.99
☐	434 11126 0	**How to Increase Your Sales to Industry**	Alfred Tack	£4.99
☐	434 11111 2	**How to Increase Your Sales by Telephone**	Alfred Tack	£4.99
☐	434 11106 6	**How to Overcome Nervous Tension and**		
		Speak Well in Public	Alfred Tack	£3.95
☐	434 11110 4	**How to Succeed as a Sales Manager**	Alfred Tack	£3.95
☐	434 11125 2	**How to Succeed in Selling**	Alfred Tack	£4.99
☐	437 95156 1	**Marketing: The Sales Manager's Role**	Alfred Tack	£3.50
☐	434 11132 5	**1000 Ways to Increase Your Sales**	Alfred Tack	£4.99
☐	434 11105 8	**The Courage to Grieve: Creative Living,**		
		Recovery and Growth, Through Grief	Judith Tatelbaum	£3.95
☐	434 11122 8	**Seeds of Greatness: the ten best-kept**		
		secrets of total success	Denis Waitley	£3.95
☐	434 98172 9	**Letters of a Businessman to His Son:**	G. Kingsley Ward	£4.99
		'The Extraordinary Book that has Changed		
		a Million Business Lives'		

Peter Grose Ltd, PO Box 18, Mayhill, Monmouth, Gwent NP5 4YD.

Please send cheque (made out to Peter Grose Ltd) or postal order, or credit card details below, for purchase price quoted and allow the following for postage and packing:

UK, BFPO & Eire	£1 for the first book, 50p for each subsequent book ordered, to a maximum charge of £2.00.
Overseas Customers	£2.00 for the first book plus 75p for each subsequent book.

NAME (Block Letters) ....

ADDRESS ....

.... Date...

VISA/ACCESS/MASTERCARD/AMERICAN EXPRESS Card No. ....

Expiry date ....

Signature ....

While every effort is made to keep prices low, it is sometimes necessary to increase prices at short notice. Cedar Books reserves the right to show new prices on covers which may differ from those previously advertised.